5-15-79

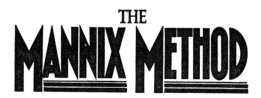

THE

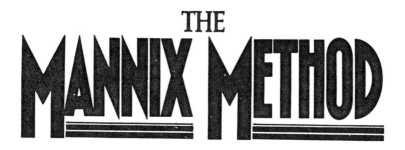

A 12-WEEK PROGRAM FOR WEIGHT CONTROL
THROUGH BEHAVIOR TRAINING

JEFFREY MANNIX

FOREWORD BY LEONARD SCHWARTZMAN, M.D.

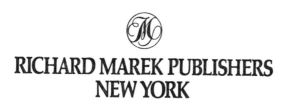

RICHARD MAREK PUBLISHERS
NEW YORK

Library of Congress Cataloging in Publication Data

Mannix, Jeffrey.
    The Mannix method.

    Includes index.
    1.   Obesity—Psychological aspects.
2.   Behavior therapy.   I.   Title.
RC552.025M36   616.3'98'06   78-31219
ISBN 0–399–90048–9

PRINTED IN THE UNITED STATES OF AMERICA.

CONTENTS

SESSION 4

SESSION 5

SESSION 6

SESSION 7

SESSION 8

SESSION 11

SESSION 12

FOREWORD

Despite the plethora of "diet books" which are readily available in a variety of shops including food markets, patients frequently consult a physician for assistance with weight reduction. Nearly all these patients present a long history of dissatisfaction with their body and body weight, frequently since childhood. Nearly all these patients secretly hope that a medical evaluation will uncover some simply corrected metabolic abnormality that will solve the weight problem, forever. Nearly all these patients are disappointed to hear what they already know, that only a modification of their eating pattern will result in a weight change.

In counseling such a patient, the physician must first evaluate the patient's general state of health, and consider whether a particular diet might provoke or complicate any underlying biochemical, physiological, or psychological disorder. Patients with diabetes, gout, hypertension, heart disease, and patients taking certain medications require special attention. This foreword, however, applies primarily to the healthy, overweight adult.

11

As a youngster at home I remember adult family members and friends "going on" the liquid, the grapefruit, and the Mayo Clinic diets. Thirty years later, as a physician in my office, I hear patients discuss going on the high protein, the liquid protein, the low carbohydrate, the drinking man's, the ski team, the Scarsdale, and still other diets. Indeed, all these diets, old and new, work. They work because they offer a brief, intense, simple and sometimes interesting exposure to reduced caloric intake. However, the therapeutic goal is not a transient, but rather a long term control of body fat, and this goal is not often achieved with these diets. In fact, the likelihood of helping a patient reach and maintain an ideal body weight is so small, that many doctors have lost enthusiasm for the standard format of presenting a printed diet and advising periodic office weigh-ins. Physicians have prescribed diet pills, thyroid pills, diuretics, hormone shots, and food supplements, but careful analysis of these agents reveals greater potential for harm than help. Diet doctors and diet centers have sprung up in many cities, but the long term benefits of these programs have not yet been impressive. In summary, many people want to lose weight, some need to, and few do.

My experience with "behavior modification" is still limited, but I am strongly interested in exploring it further, especially as a result of reading this work. However, several recent medical studies suggest this modality as a major advance over the usual diet regimens in the treatment of obesity. I read *The Mannix Method* with increasing interest through the twelve-week program. Although some of the biochemical and physiological information presented is still controversial, the Mannix Method itself is a fascinating and revolutionary approach to the field of weight reduction. There is no doubt that the serious reader who follows the guidelines outlined in this book, step by step, incorporating each new technique of the Mannix Method of behavior training into his life-style, can indeed conquer compulsive overeating safely and permanently.

I welcome this original contribution to the field.

LEONARD SCHWARTZMAN, M.D.
Diplomate, American Board of Internal Medicine. Assistant Clinical Professor, UCLA Center for the Health Sciences. Attending Physician, Cedars–Sinai Medical Center, Los Angeles, California.

PREVIEW

FIRST OF ALL

Losing weight is easy. Probably everyone who is reading this book knows many, many methods and secrets for losing unwanted pounds. All theories boil down to one simple formula: Eat less than you burn up. Well, you have been trying to do just that through 17,290 publicly recorded methods to reduce weight, and it just doesn't work! Inherent in all diets is the necessity of restricting food intake. Whether you restrict food intake through counting calories and carbohydrates, increasing or limiting protein, fasting, using appetite-depressing drugs, or any other manipulation of food, you are doomed to failure before you start. There is no need to document the staggeringly high failure rate in dieting. If you yourself aren't sufficient proof, I'm sure that you know many people who have tried all the popular methods each year and are equipped once again to try the latest diet rage each new season.

It is time to face the facts and stop deluding yourself. If you want to lose weight and keep it off, you must examine closely the method you used to get fat. Then, in a systematic relearning approach, develop methods of eating that will discourage gaining

15

more body weight than your frame can handle attractively. Once you get on a realistic program of eating, and can depend on your eating behavior to keep you on that program, you will lose those excess pounds. I repeat: If you examine closely the eating habits that produced your unnecessary weight, learn behavior that will produce healthy eating attitudes, and adhere to your new behavior until it becomes dependable, you will lose excess weight at a sensible rate with no inclination to regain unwanted and unhealthy fat.

My clients are not on diets. They take no drugs. They neither count calories nor carbohydrates, nor do they weigh their foods. There is no prescribed exercise, no trick food, no attempt to fool the stomach. My clients are on a program of learning to eat sensibly, and in doing so begin to understand how to gain pleasure in other ways than eating. You too can end a nightmarish fight with weight. *You can end it if you want to and are ready now.*

FIND THE FACTS

Be prepared to discover your *real* reasons for wanting to change.

When clients come to the Mannix Clinic, I always ask, "Why do you want to lose weight?"

They all laugh and reply that it seems quite obvious. But it is not obvious. Being fat is not a reason to lose weight. Losing weight is not a goal in itself, but a path to that goal.

Stop right now and list three of your most important reasons for wanting to lose weight. Everyone's fourth reason is that he/she is finally *fed up with fat.*

1. _____

_____

2. _____

_____

3. _____

_____

4. _____

_____

If one or two of your reasons for wanting to be thin are important enough to sustain your effort throughout this twelve-week training, the Mannix Method will change your life.

WHY ME?

Children are taught to overeat. Your eating behavior is learned. Abusive eating habits have caused your condition. But no matter how you trace back to causes, you are schooled in overeating. And face one thing: It's your behavior, and only you can change it. Your path, your present direction, significantly increases your chances of developing diabetes, strokes, heart attacks, high blood pressure, digestive disease, kidney disease, gallbladder malfunctions, skin problems, back problems, joint diseases, varicose veins, emphysema, and scores of other less crippling conditions that create the stress necessary to shorten an uncomfortable life.

Make up your mind that you are finished with fat. You are finished with this obsession with the food that controls you. It is time to take responsibility for reversing conditions. It doesn't take willpower, or some enormous strength that you lack. You just don't know how to use your strengths. You have been stuck for so long out of control that you are probably confused and afraid. You have been disappointed and discouraged with diets, and maybe even more recently with hypnosis and medication. But if you are willing to try to lose weight just one more time, it can be done *easily, permanently,* and *with dignity.*

It is a myth that the weight reducer can achieve his goals alone. The person who goes it alone without a plan or a method pits himself against all of the forces that have created his problem. It is a process that takes time, sustained attention, sincere desire, and a helping hand.

WHAT'S THE DEAL?

There is one idea basic to this book: You are fat and less attractive than you can be, and you are doing it to yourself. Of all possible escapes or vices or self-indulgences, you chose eating. You'd like to be let off the hook. Your problem is not food, it is eating. The only reason that you are fat is that you eat too much too frequently, and you eat the wrong foods. One more thing: Only you can do something about it. It's good to ask for help. As a matter of fact it's the only thing to do. You've tried it alone, and don't need to be reminded of the dismal results. You made the first move when you bought this book. Now, stay on the track. I believe that you have always wanted to do something about your condition. Most overweight people know more about nutrition and calories than many doctors. Understand completely that alternatives to control are just deception. You are not fooling anyone and are wasting time in conflict. You can't deceive any longer with your blouse out or your collars wide. A bubbling personality and personal sacrifices don't cover up, either. Fat is unhealthy and disabling. And in a complex way, the people around you may contribute to your fat. That may sound cruel, but it may be very possible.

There is no doubt that there are underlying causes for overindulgence. You will find them as you proceed to uncover the real you from under all that tissue. First, however, let's alter behavior so you may begin to enjoy the rewards of being free of ugly fat and in control of your life.

The most important item in the deal is what you have to do to make it all possible. It will take some effort, but hundreds of people just like you have done it. You must simply take responsibility for your condition and commit yourself, with each new session, to practicing the simple outlined steps. Don't permit any self-consciousness to hamper your success.

There is a contract at the end of each session for you to initial if you are willing to contract for seven days of conscientious practice. Sign the contract! Obligate yourself in writing! The act of signing will commit you to one session at a time. If you are conscientious and live up to your pledged word, you will move on to the next session with a greater degree of mastery.

After working through all of the sessions, a young and very attractive client was reviewing her experiences and behavior changes, which resulted in a loss of forty pounds. We were discussing how her life goals and expectations had changed substantially. She had developed skills for responding to early signals that need attention in maintaining desired eating habits. At the end of one of our meetings, I asked her if, in retrospect, she thought the Mannix Method difficult. "You know," she said, "I take piano lessons two and sometimes three times a week. I've been studying for almost five years now. It has never failed that when my teacher introduces me to a new and more demanding piece of music, I look at the first page and exclaim that I can't possibly handle such an intricate assignment. I'm always positively sure that this time he has really overestimated my capabilities. I look back at five years of that kind of resistance and I laugh at myself for having been afraid of each new challenge, knowing how easily I can handle them all."

Systematically changing your behavior will train you to redirect your efforts comfortably, one step at a time. Read each session and follow the training methods exactly as they are presented, and for the required time. Remember that you are free to stop after completing any session, if you wish. But while you are participating, be precise. Do not pick and choose the way you will practice these procedures. If you spend just one third of the time you now use to work at being fat working at this method of losing fat instead, you will control your weight and change your appearance with ease.

ON YOUR MARK

For eight weeks you will be keeping a Food Journal. This journal will become a record of everything that you eat every day. To fix your starting position, you will keep a baseline Food Journal for the next seven days. Starting tomorrow morning, record everything you eat in the Journal, filling in each column. This baseline eating record is private, so don't be embarrassed or withhold any entry because you may think that the small amount of some snack is unimportant, or that you swallowed it too fast for it to matter. Record every morsel that passes your lips. Record all beverages with the exception of water. Include diet sodas, alcohol, juice, coffee, and tea.

The purpose of this one-week baseline Food Journal is to make you completely aware of your current eating habits, with full knowledge of amounts and frequencies, so that you may begin to discover some of your reasons for eating. Chances are that most of your eating is in response to external cues like the time of day, television commercials, the smell of food, the sight of friends, or just the overavailability of food, rather than the internal cue of hunger. You must begin to gain some insight into cues, because they trigger the response behavior you use to overeat. In the column labeled ATTITUDE, be sure to record your mood while eating. My clients write one of the following words in that column:

Relaxed
Agitated
Angry
Bored

Next to the word that best describes your attitude while eating, try to evaluate your degree of hunger. Use 0 to indicate no hunger, 1 for slight hunger, 2 for moderate hunger, and 3 for hungry.

Use as many lines as are necessary, and more than one page for each day if you need to. Be meticulous with your Journal. It is not punishment. It is a tool for gathering information about you—for you. As you proceed from Session 1, you will be able to refer back to this baseline Journal to plot your progress and to analyze it for insights and patterns.

Right is an example of a completed page of a baseline Journal:

Food Journal

In the appendix you will find a blank Food Journal page designed to be easily reproduced by any photocopying machine. Just take the entire book to an instant press or quick copy store and they will be able to run off as many pages of the blank Journal page as you need. The blank Journal page is sized so that it can be inserted into a pocket or purse size checkbook cover. If you reproduce twenty copies of the blank Journal page, then trim and staple the pages together, you can fit more than two week's worth into your checkbook cover and always be assured of having an available and well ordered Food Journal. If a photocopy machine is not available to you, simply purchase a small spiral-bound pocket notebook and rule off the columns and entry spaces using the blank Journal page as a guide.

As soon as you have decided upon a method that suits you best, begin carrying your Food Journal with you wherever you

DATE	START TIME	FOOD/AMOUNT	ATTITUDE	FINISH TIME	TOTAL EATING TIME
Sun 12th	8:30 AM	2 eggs, 2 bacon, 1 toast	Relaxed 1	8:42 AM	12
	9:10 AM	1 toast with peanut butter	Bored 2	9:15 AM	5
	9:30 AM	1 cup coffee—cream, 2 sugar	Bored 3	9:40 AM	10
	11:30 AM	1 tuna sandwich, small bag of potato chips, 1 8-oz. milk	Agitated 2	11:45 AM	15
	2:00 PM	1 can root beer 1 handful of potato chips	Angry 3	2:20 PM	20
	3:30 PM	½ peanut & jelly sandwich	Angry 3	3:35 PM	5
	3:35 PM	2 oatmeal cookies 1 8-oz. milk	Angry 3	3:37 PM	2
	6:00 PM	1 8-oz. cocktail—rye & ginger	Relaxed 3	6:18 PM	18
	6:30 PM	1 8-oz. cocktail—rye & ginger	Relaxed 2	7:00 PM	30
	7:00 PM	B-B-Qed steak, french fries, small dinner salad	Relaxed 2	7:15 PM	15
	7:30 PM	1 lg. piece *homemade* cho. cake	Relaxed 1	7:35 PM	5
	9:10 PM	Approx. 20 peanuts (watching TV)	Relaxed 3	9:11 PM	1
	10:00 PM	1 piece cho. cake	Agitated 3	10:10 PM	10
	11:30 PM	"pinch" of cake—8 oz. milk	Tired	11:31 PM	1
Mon 13th	7:05 AM	1 English muffin—butter & cream cheese	Agitated 2	7:15 AM	10
	7:30 AM	1 cup coffee—cream & 2 sugar	Agitated 3	7:45 AM	15
	7:45 AM	2 oatmeal cookies LATE FOR WORK—out the door!	Agitated 1	7:50 AM	5
	10:00 AM	Coffee break—1 donut 1 coffee	Bored	10:10 AM	10

go. If you leave it behind by accident one day, write down everything you eat on a separate slip of paper and enter everything in the Food Journal as soon as you get back to it. If it does happen that you forget your Food Journal, make a point of placing it in a more conspicuous place the next day; perhaps under your keys or with your pocket money. It might take some extra thought to carry it with you for the first few days, but if you are conscientious about it, remembering to include it along with your personal belongings will quickly become automatic.

HABIT AWARENESS

The object of this program is to teach you to eat in a way that will lead to permanent weight *control* with your weight loss. You must be interested in weight loss only as a result of behavior change. The primary reason diets, pills, and shots are ineffective is that their use must be limited. When the diet or the drug is finished, most people resume their familiar old patterns of eating and rapidly regain every ounce of fat.

You must establish priorities to control your eating habits. If losing weight, resolving your compulsion for food, and gaining control of your life are important to you, you will definitely succeed. It takes time and calculated effort. It is not like stopping a locomotive. It requires stick-to-it-iveness and deliberation. Through each and every session, you will learn simple procedures to practice, so deceptively simple that they may seem to contribute little to your overall goals. But combine all of the simple skills you are practicing, and your goals will always be in view, your progress will be steady, and your life will improve with each day of pleasant repetition. You will lose one or two pounds per week. Remember, it was a slow process to gain your excess weight, so don't permit yourself to be impatient losing it. You are not on a diet. You must eat your way back to your normal size if you expect to remain there, and it must take time. Once again, you are not merely trying to lose weight, you are learning to change your behavior. You are learning to change the eating and thinking patterns that distort your body and your mind.

No matter how much weight you need to lose, your most important goal is to learn management of your eating. It will improve everything in your life. Be prepared to climb out of the dark and shadowy side of life and get ready to experience varied and exciting new pleasures. Get ready to leave behind you the obsessive attention that you pay to yourself and to your problems. As you master control and you lose weight, enjoy it! Branch out! Try new experiences. Meet new people. Go places as you lose your self-consciousness. Fill your mind with "other-directed" thoughts. You might even begin a slow reevaluation of your fat friends. As your attitude about yourself changes, your environment will follow right along. Your activities will no longer need to be geared for the partially handicapped. Consequently, the other actors in your play might have to be recast to add cheer and optimism to your world instead of the usual discouragement and envy.

You have probably known a few people who managed to diet away a sizeable amount of fat and to maintain the loss for a few months. I've met some of those "thin-fat" people. They spend more time than they ever did, working on food-restrictive gimmicks and special recipes and concoctions. They are haunted with the horror of ever eating and ballooning up again. They know no peace. Eating has become the single most important activity in their lives. These thin-fat people have developed normal weight. They don't look fat anymore—except in their own minds. They are as fat and obsessed with thoughts of food as they ever were. That kind of confusion has to lead to some kind of disorientation, or at best a desperate perceptual conflict. No one can be blamed for gaining back the weight lost on a diet—it's a natural phenomenon. You must either grow fat again or go mad staying thin. We respond to signals without being aware of those signals. It is certainly obvious that your instinctive mind comes to the rescue and arranges ways for you to get fat again, if there is the slightest danger that your new thin condition threatens your usual you—your familiar identity. Simple diets don't work because the food didn't make you fat—your eating patterns did.

Behavior modification goals are designed to be permanent. They are designed to replace previously inappropriate ways of doing things. If much of your activity is performed with undesirable behavior, learn to redesign it . . . learn to change. Don't dare this method to help you! Understand the techniques and look for ways to help yourself. You will change your eating behavior and that will, in turn, affect your feelings about food. By regulating the action, which is controlled directly by your perception, you can regulate your feelings indirectly. You act as you change your point of view.

Time is important, or at least the use of time. You will be taking more time to eat than you do now, so that you learn to experience food thoughtfully and enjoy it thoroughly. If you can't spare the time to experience eating, you may achieve less than your best on this program.

Your first job is to develop habit awareness. You will examine your present eating habits in detail, and you will discover the specific behaviors that reinforced your weight problem. Once you have identified those behaviors, you will proceed to determine which environmental factors control those behaviors. With that information, you will be able to make changes in your environment that will support the new behavior patterns you are working for.

Changing any habit takes continuous attention and determination. Don't make the mistake of trying to handle more than you are capable of, at first. That will invite failure. The way to succeed is to take small steps, and to practice each step until it is overlearned. It then becomes a habit—an almost automatic action. Impatience to hurry with this program or to hasten your weight loss will set you up for failure. This is not the time to demonstrate your fast learning ability. And do not move through this program judging your own pace. Trust the process and *follow the instructions precisely,* and you will win the biggest and best prize that you have ever bargained for.

Begin thinking about just what your priorities are in this adventure. Think about them before you start the program. Perhaps you may decide that taking time to prepare and eat breakfast isn't as important to you as that time spent in bed. It may be that spending those extra minutes in bed in the morning is just as important to you as losing weight. Perhaps pizza and beer after bowling are more important to you right now than losing weight. There may be a number of priorities that you place before your need to effect behavior change to lose weight. Be fully aware of your options. Be responsible for your choices. Change requires sustained effort—it is a process, not an event—and you will be successful only if you understand that. Short-term losses are relatively unimportant. To make this program work for you, you must know basic first principles now and new ideas as they are introduced. After you understand and apply each technique, you must practice it until it is a habit. You must always be sensitive to habits that may become lazy, permitting those old destructive patterns to take over. Appropriate eating is a valuable lifetime skill that is practiced by anyone you know who is healthy.

Please be aware, too, that you have developed the habit of substance abuse. You can change the behavior that led to that abuse if you recognize that you possess the ability to abuse the particular substance called food. It is very much like the reformed alcoholic knowing that he/she abuses alcohol, particularly when offered a glass of wine or beer. You will always have to be practicing your new food management skills. Occasionally you must just plain discipline your behavior for the moment to exercise control, when temptation, the "just this once," is pounding in your ears at a special party or football game or any gathering around food. Abusive eating is nothing less than addiction.

AVOID UNACCUSTOMED EXERCISE

The idea of an overweight person planning and sticking to a rigorous program of exercise is preposterous. Unaccustomed physical exertion expended now for some poorly defined reward in six months, or in the vague future, must be doomed to failure by its own design. One of the shared characteristics of individuals with an eating problem is their obvious inability to postpone pleasure. Your feeling of well-being and abundant energy must evolve from a pleasant and agreeable source of movement. Vigorous exercise is for the physically fit, and carrying excess weight makes you physically unfit. It is a conflict of interests. Interest in the immediate pleasure of eating has become more important than the promise of things to come, especially the promise of an abstract thing like a feeling of well-being that has never been experienced. It took a long time to make those extra pounds a structural part of your body, and it took that much time again to recognize that the fat was not going to disappear by itself. Add to that "fat" time the time spent on at least one diet. What might have been a casual weight gain has turned into a major lifetime disappointing struggle, laden with feelings of guilt and failure.

Please do not begin an exercise program until you have achieved a good degree of eating control with success. Exercise is uncommon among average-sized people. Consider exercise, vigorous exercise—out.

During our stepping up of commitments, you will be asked to manage a walk every day. It is necessary for you to experience pleasure from appropriate behavior. As you lose weight and gain control of your health, walk to relax and feel every part of your body moving you along.

As your developing new eating habits result in more energy and a continuing loss of weight, you will probably want to increase your physical activity. Longer walks may be the next step. Or you may want to explore more active things. In any event, avoid the idea of isolated exercise, at least for a few months.

YOU ARE ONE

It is now time to realize that the mind and the body are one living entity with myriad parts that function differently and separately, but in harmony. The health of the body and its organs is completely dependent on the health of the mind. A variety of foods in your diet supplies the slightly different fuels that each organ needs to function best. These organs interact to create a condition of health. The healthy condition of the mind also affects body functions. *Everything* interacts. You supply the proper fuel for every part of your body, including fuel for the mind. The mind is fueled by special nutrients supplied from food, but it also needs a fuel that it manufactures for itself. The mind's extra fuel requirement is reward. Rewards are appraised with the mind. You must feed the receptive and reward-seeking mind function to make use of the Mannix Method of weight control. The mind and the body work together to create harmony. The mind function is the most important part of your retraining. So begin the first session with the personal commitment to "reach beyond your grasp."

You will practice behavior modification on the functions of both the body and the mind. Notice improvement in your health as soon as you begin, and compliment yourself when you succeed. Enjoy all of your food, reward yourself with occasional gifts for not disappointing yourself, and try, with all your being, to see the forest as a group of trees. Help yourself to succeed. My clients succeed because they commit themselves to one step at a time, and they develop faith in themselves and their ability to change. They know that they can succeed, and are willing to sign contracts with themselves. They promise themselves—not me, nor the guy next door. You will do just that when you initial the contract for each session as you work on the program in this book. Give yourself a chance. Be careful not to overcommit. Work at the pace set with each new session. You can make it all the way, if you can continue to fuel all of your mind/body functions properly. Take charge and make the start.

TWENTY-ONE DAYS TO NEW HABITS

Behavior modification is no more complicated than learning new behavior and practicing that new behavior until it becomes dominant. The emphasis here is on *practice*. New patterns of behaving must be practiced for at least twenty-one days to make them trustworthy. The substance is not the culprit. Food is not the problem; eating it is the problem. Overeating, or abusive eating, can only be unlearned and replaced with selective eating patterns that are practiced continuously. You must practice the skills taught in each session before going on to the following session. Each new session will introduce new skills.

You are about to alter present activities by learning to substitute and to prefer alternate activities. Appreciate the significance of the undertaking. In order to be fully successful, plan to change your taste for heavy, rich, or sweet foods to the more healthful lighter foods that are less fattening and more nourishing. That's a large order deserving of your full attention when dealing with food. The only way that you can effect such a change in taste and behavior is to want to change. No one can force this on you. None of us can tolerate rules and regulations imposed on us. But if we are permitted to share in formulating the rules and regulations, we feel personally responsible for the guidelines and will choose to follow them.

PRIORITIES

Make your weight control top priority in your life right now. A few weeks of high-priority status now will eliminate a disabling preoccupation with future misery day after day. What a joy it can be to use your days for pleasurable activity and to fill your thoughts with hope. Not only will you succeed in losing unwanted pounds, but you will be succeeding in accepting yourself, perhaps for the first time in your life. You will actually like yourself. My clients realize that when they gain control over food so they look and feel better, everything in every area of their lives benefits from the overflow. Confidence comes hand in hand with your self-image. Why not reexamine all the situations in your life—your marriage, your job, relationships, hobbies, your favorite colors, your hairstyle, everything. Be freshly aware of everything. If the other situations are working well for you and are giving you a feeling of satisfaction, they will not suffer from close examination. If they are outdated and just useless baggage, now is the perfect time to recognize their drain on you and to prepare to make some changes. Examine the rituals that you have become so secure and comfortable with. Chances are you will discover more than one that is no longer rewarding or useful. Many may be actually punitive. Don't approach this program timidly—be aggressive. Insist on the right to alter your environment for your well-being. Work yourself out of self-made traps. You are not the victim of your condition; you can be the master and change it. Do it now, and be prepared to let go of anything that keeps you immobilized to your disadvantage. You are about to open the doors to a world that is new and exciting. Just the peace of mind achieved with controlling your weight will produce reward enough to encourage you to reject the momentary pleasure of overeating. Your body movements will reflect the way you feel inside. You will be able to dress in any style that delights you. You will be proud of your self-discipline and your ability to do what you set your mind to. You will end the ever-present shame and self-consciousness you have been living with until now. Underneath all of your fat there is a vital, a beautiful you. Find that other person. Live your life, and the time is now!

You are now going to begin the training sessions. There are a few points that you want to have fixed in your mind before you start. It is time to decide about the significance of change. Don't postpone that decision. Make it now, knowing that you are planning to alter the path your life has taken so far.

Diets do not work. Period. They are great for taking weight off time and time again, but they hinder more than they help with permanently controlling your weight. The Mannix Method is not a way to reduce, but rather a process for learning the use of techniques that prevent unhealthy fat. There is little sense in just restricting food to lose weight. You will automatically regain those pounds of fat when the diet time is expired. You will now lose weight simply as a by-product of changing the way you behave with food. You are going to deal with the source of the problem, not the surface symptoms.

Your commitment to proceed through the sessions is your choice. This is a program designed to change your behavior. Remember that it takes at least twenty-one repetitions of a performance to incorporate new behavior. Twenty-one days of practicing this new program will develop dependable new habits that will give you the confidence to control every facet of your life! Twenty-one days of practicing without variation, and with enthusiasm, will produce enough feeling of well-being to sustain your determination. You will lose pounds easily and you will change your self-destructive behavior. This theme is repeated in a number of different ways, with the hope that the scheme is impressively clear. You will change the way you use food and think about food, so that you may relieve your body of all excess fat permanently. Food itself is not the issue—eating is the issue. Your behavior with food is what it is all about!

This program does not dictate what to eat, nor is it a medical program. But any change in routine benefits if it is preceded by a thorough physical checkup by your family doctor or internist.

SESSION 1

FOOD FOR THOUGHT

Have you ever stopped to realize that we are not plugged in at night like golf carts, nor do we have a power source to which we are connected with long cords, nor do we swallow some kind of magic potion or periodically inject a fluid to keep us running? Food is our fuel. Food is our source of energy. The careful selection and proper administration of food determines our life condition. Think of the enormity of that fact for a moment. Here we are, completely involved with taste treats and chemical additives to please the palate, when our most pressing concern should be the effective fueling of our life machinery. Certainly, we have lost sight of the basic facts. The most delicate, and consequently the most easily damaged, cells in our bodies are the cells of the brain. Improper nourishment of brain cells—our command-center cells, so to speak—results in the poor management of the total body. We must, therefore, meet the requirements of the brain before we can hope to control the health of the body.

Blood sugar (glucose) is the fuel for the brain and the source of energy for the body. A meager supply of fuel to the brain produces serious stress. Depression is a necessary mental consequence of a low-blood-sugar condition in the brain. Many ill-informed psychiatric patients could relieve depression by altering their diets to correct the imbalance of blood sugar. Fatigue is also a consequence of insufficient fueling for high energy demand.

Following is a list of some of the more common symptoms of low blood sugar. Of course, your doctor should be consulted, because many of these symptoms may indicate a variety of malfunctions. However, low blood sugar should be considered suspect when any of these conditions accompany excess fat:

dizzy spells	anxiety
headaches	depression
undue fatigue	attacks of weakness
feeling of exhaustion	light-headedness
drowsiness	without fainting
muscular pain	tremors,
leg cramps	cold sweating
insomnia	inner trembling
nervousness	poor concentration
rapid heart action	convulsions
lack of coordination	blurred vision

Low blood sugar, or hypoglycemia, is not a disease. It represents, for the most part, a regulatory dysfunction of the body. Overeating, poor food choice, and long periods of fasting have confused the sugar-regulating function. For the person trying to lose weight, low blood sugar is a double threat. It not only makes you feel depressed, it also makes you feel hungry. The more you eat, the more insulin you produce and the sooner you want to eat again. It's a vicious cycle that must be interrupted long enough to restructure your eating patterns to promote the proper mixture of insulin and sugar in the blood.

When you awaken in the morning, your blood sugar is at the fasting level. If you have a cup of coffee and a doughnut for breakfast, the sugar and starch carbohydrates in the doughnut and the caffeine in the coffee may possibly send your blood sugar skyrocketing. Somewhere in that upward thrust, insulin is called for, acting immediately to force the blood sugar level down to a safe mixture. Because the doughnut and coffee have no real food

value, the force of the insulin cannot be resisted. The blood sugar
is then reduced to a point that is lower than the original fasting
level. That is why, after an instant morning burst of energy, an
hour or so later, you usually experience some of the symptoms of
low blood sugar. When blood glucose is driven to an extremely
low level, the brain is being starved and the body runs ineffi-
ciently. You cannot lose weight without a respectable blood glucose level. You certainly can never control eating when your fuel
supply is depleted most of the time and then indiscriminately replenished. (See *Body, Mind, and Sugar* by Dr. E. M. Abraham-
son.)   C872540

Low blood sugar stresses the body. The stress response, and
the behavior related to this biochemical adjustment, are involved
in overeating and overdrinking. The results of low blood sugar
can be devastating.

Caffeine in coffee, tea, cola, and chocolate stimulates the brain
to produce more hormones. The hormones stimulate the liver to
release glucose into the bloodstream. The freshly sugar-enriched
blood calls for insulin, but as with the morning coffee and
doughnut, if there is no other food in the system there is no substance to fend off the force of the insulin. So the blood sugar
plummets. Anyone using these caffeine products to fight hunger
or to increase energy is compounding an already bad condition.
It is sensible to discontinue the use of caffeine in your diet, including artificially sweetened cola.

One last point before beginning Session 1. Sugar is a substance
that should be avoided like the plague. For many of you, sugar is
the major reason for extra weight. The thought of abstaining
from sugary treats may frighten you. I see many clients who are
truly "hooked" on sugar. I believe that sugar may be addictive,
usually leading to compulsive eating of sweets. Candy, cake, or
cookie binges are common among many obese people. Again,
this develops as the result of dangerously low blood sugar and a
stress response that must be interrupted long enough for the metabolism to level off. The liberal use of fresh fruit in your eating
plans will help the withdrawal from refined sugar. If your body
has a need for the stimulating effects of sugar, fruit will satisfy
that need without the damaging side effects.

Sugar is poison, make no mistake about that. With the Mannix

Method you can slowly eliminate sugar from your diet with little difficulty.

Now, begin Session 1 of the Mannix Method of Weight Control. This Method is for you to use to improve your total person, affecting your total existence. This Method has been tested and used with enormous success. It will lead you to a better understanding of everything in your environment, in addition to a complete understanding of your eating patterns. Good luck! Be strong! Be assertive! Be patient! Be you at your very best!

TAPERED EATING

Tapered eating provides appropriate foods at each meal to meet the fuel demands of your body for best energy output. Breakfast is the largest and most important meal of your day. Lunch is very important, but should be smaller in volume. Supper is the least important meal as far as your body needs for fuel are concerned, and should therefore be the lightest meal of your day. Also, eat no food for four hours before going to sleep.

This sequence of food intake is probably the reverse of your usual pattern. For many of you, this will be the first time in a long time that you will be eating whole meals. For some—those of you who already eat breakfast regularly—this tapering style is easy to grasp. No matter how your eating habits compare to this procedure, for only twelve weeks it is imperative that you schedule your day to include these three meals in the described descending order of volume and fuel value.

Food selection and portion size are left to your discretion. The amount of food that you eat and the variety of the foods that you choose are left entirely up to you. There are few overweight people who don't know precisely which foods are "fattening" and what portion sizes are gluttonous. These areas are your responsibility. However, select the best foods you can find and prepare them in the most nutritious ways. If you must use canned food, check the labels to make sure that the ingredients do not include sugar and unnecessary additives. It is also advisable for you to eat fresh fruit and fresh vegetables whenever you can get them. They have the most nutritional value and are far more exciting to prepare than dull canned and packaged foods.

Tapered Eating, or energy/demand eating, looks like the following diagram:

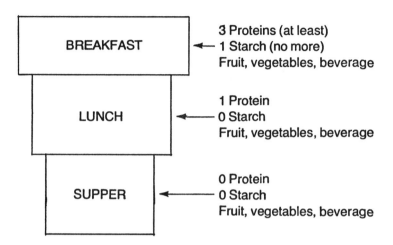

BREAKFAST ← 3 Proteins (at least)
1 Starch (no more)
Fruit, vegetables, beverage

LUNCH ← 1 Protein
0 Starch
Fruit, vegetables, beverage

SUPPER ← 0 Protein
0 Starch
Fruit, vegetables, beverage

No food for at least four hours before retiring.
Include vegetables, fruit, and beverages with an eye to calories.

Breakfast

The BANQUET of the day! Eat anything that you may have wanted for dinner last night.
1. This is the largest meal of your day.
2. Eat three proteins. Eat more proteins if you anticipate a long or an active day.
3. Proteins: One protein is a typical serving of:
    meat
    fish
    dairy products—cheese, yogurt, eggs
    poultry
    nuts
    vegetable protein—avocado, soy products
4. Eat only one starch—select toast or bread as your starch, with butter if you like your toast buttered. Have two slices, if you wish, although one slice serves your goals better. BUT: Do not permit yourself to feel deprived. Other

starches are potatoes, pasta, corn bread, pizza, or cake if you must.
5. Beverage
6. Fruit and vegetables

Lunch

Don't skip it; this is a very important meal.
1. This is your second-largest meal of the day.
2. Eat one protein—two are permissible for active schedules.
3. Eat no starch—of course sandwiches will have to be saved for your breakfast.
4. Beverage if you wish.
5. Fruit and vegetables—if you wish.

Supper

This is the least important meal of the day for energy output.
1. This is probably the meal that has been responsible for much of your fat. You can't go to bed with a full stomach and expect to control your weight!
2. No protein.
3. No starch.
4. Salads and vegetables get top billing here. Lighter salad dressings give you the edge. Invest in a good vegetarian cookbook. The recipes are exciting, the creations delicious and healthy. Save proteins and starch, or birthday cake (occasional), for breakfast.

Evening Snacks

This snacking is Enemy #1.
1. The food that you eat directly before you go to bed will turn to fat while you sleep, and will confuse your control systems in the morning.
2. Night eating is all habit and no hunger.
3. This habit will be the easiest habit to break, if it is not reinforced for a very few nights. If you think that you are hungry, which is highly improbable, drink a glass of water and

go to sleep while visions of breakfast treats dance in your head. Plan an irresistible menu. An empty stomach and relaxed digestive apparatus will contribute to restful sleep. You will awaken revitalized! So, please, no food four hours before bed!

Becoming thin in the process of becoming healthy means that the only way to regain lost pounds is to become unhealthy once again. It has been proved over and over again that every living thing does its best to improve its condition and to grow toward optimal health. It seems that only poor environmental conditions alter this natural tendency for improvement. Poor environmental conditions caused you to overeat to become fat. You can buck almost any destructive outside influence by deciding to follow your natural instinct for improvement. The Mannix Method is precisely an outline for self-improvement.

The fear of change can be overpowering, so follow your instinct for self-improvement and trust this method. It is all plain common sense. Records in my office prove that you will lose unnecessary weight by supplying your body with the proper food at the times that it is needed most. After a long period of unconscious rest, just before a long period of demanding activity, your body needs nourishment (breakfast time). During any period of extended activity, your body demands additional fuel (lunchtime), and as activity diminishes, the body requires little more than rest (suppertime).

You must meet the basic fuel requirements of the body machine.

INTRODUCTION TO THE FOOD JOURNAL

The single most important tool that you will use throughout these learning sessions is the Food Journal. The Journal has two main conditions, and you must understand them before you are able to use your Journal information. First, the Journal must be used to record *everything* that you eat. Second, the Journal must be used *before* you eat anything. The key words are: *what* and *when*. The accuracy of your records will make the use of your recorded information easier.

Simply then:

1. The Food Journal is a *record* of *what* you are eating.
2. The Food Journal is *not* a *confession* of what you ate.
3. The Food Journal makes you *aware* of what you eat *before* you eat it.
4. Everything counts, including that "little taste" of something that you didn't plan to eat.
5. The Food Journal serves you best if it is *accurate.*

If you miss the point that the Journal is a record of what you are eating, and *not* a confession of what you ate, you will reinforce the dieter's familiar guilt pattern. You will retard your progress. This record takes some effort, and if you go to the trouble of recording at all, recognize that the effort produces the best results when you *write before you eat.* This will prove significantly valuable as the weeks go on.

KEEPING THE FOOD JOURNAL

The Food Journal is vitally important to give you immediate feedback about what and when you eat. Please be accurate, honest, and enthusiastic. Plunge into this effort with a spirit of acceptance and adventure.

1. Record the day and date on the top of each page.
2. Use as many pages as necessary for each day. Resist economizing; elaborate.
3. Write legibly and in detail.
4. Record the *time* that you begin to eat, the *food* that you are about to eat, the approximate *portions* of food. Record *all* of this information *before* you sit down to eat. (Preplanned menus are great but not required.)
5. *After* you have eaten, check the clock again and put the hour in the FINISH TIME column.
6. Record your feelings in the column marked ATTITUDE. Use the following descriptive words:
Relaxed
Agitated
Angry
Bored
7. You needn't continue to rate degree of hunger. If, however, you find that information beneficial, by all means continue.

You will discover a great deal about the eating situations in your life when you describe your feelings. Patterns will emerge. You may find that breakfast is your most quiet and peaceful meal. Perhaps you will be alone and unhurried, with the time to think and to develop your own special environment. Supper may emerge as your most restless meal. Maybe your lunchtime is filled with unbelievable pressure for you to meet time restrictions. Be thoughtful with your assessment of your feelings. The information gathered from that column may be the most important insight that you will gain from the entire Journal. Feel free to add comments to your Food Journal any time you think further explanation might lend insight.

BEHAVIOR RULES

Your work with the Mannix Method involves the practice or repetition of a set of actions that you will use every time you are involved with food. No one of these actions is difficult, but each one must be given sufficient time to develop into a reliable habit. It must, therefore, be practiced honestly, leaving no room for failure. If any task in this session, or any other session, seems too demanding, postpone it until the following session, or until you gain the confidence to complete it without failure. However, be assured that no task should prove too difficult. Each task has been designed to build on your developing ability. Practice it for the specified time, and you will become skilled in its application very quickly.

RULE 1

Write Before You Eat.
The Food Journal is your most valuable tool in learning to control your eating habits. It is easy to keep, but remember that it must be kept precisely.

RULE 2

Eat Only at Appropriate Eating Places.
Make sure that everything you eat is eaten at a place that you have reserved for eating only. You may decide to designate vari-

ous eating places as appropriate, but those places may not be used for any other activities. Breakfast may be at your kitchen table, lunch at a restaurant table, and supper at your dining-room table. Do not eat in the den or while sitting on the living-room couch, or in bed, or in your car. And never, ever, eat while you are standing up. Eating must be a deliberate, thoughtful activity. If you are the cook and you sample the food in the pot, take that sample over to the kitchen table and sit down to really taste it.

If efficiency is the style of your living quarters, and one surface serves as a work table or desk and also serves as your dining table, set all work aside where you won't be tempted by it. Turn the surface into a dining table by always using a table mat dressed with napkin and flatware. Set the dining table before you sit down to dine so that you can arrive just to eat. At the end of your meal, undress and rearrange the table before you return to work.

The application of this rule, combined with logging good records in your Food Journal, will begin to tell you almost everything there is to know about your eating habits. Nothing will escape your scientific observation, and you will begin to understand the concept of *control.*

Too often in the life of the overweight person, eating is cued by external stimuli and not by the internal need to satisfy hunger. Frequently, just walking in the front door is the cue to go to the kitchen to eat. You will learn to eliminate all those external eating cues and to develop the habit of responding only to the inner real need to satisfy hunger. By insisting that you eat only at an appropriate eating place every time you eat, you will become aware of the external cues that secretly work to make you eat. The awareness and analysis of the artificial cues that trigger your eating contribute to your ability to develop resistance to those cues. By adhering to the rule of eating only at designated eating places, you will give yourself the opportunity and the time to decide, *before* you eat anything, whether or not you are really hungry or you are just trapped in a chain-of-behavior response to an artificial cue. What's more, you will learn that eating without true hunger is not really very satisfying.

RULE 3

Eat Only; Perform No Other Activity When You Eat.

This rule of behavior follows right along with the previous rule of eating only at an appropriate eating place. DO NOT do anything else while you are eating. This means that you DO NOT watch television, DO NOT read, DO NOT talk on the phone, and DO NOT write while you eat. The goal here is for you to give your undivided attention to your food while you eat it. If you perform some additional activity when you eat, you dissipate your concentration and you will not fully appreciate your food.

Contrary to what seems to be the obvious, overweight individuals don't really like food. They abuse that particular substance and the result is *fear* of food rather than *love* for food. Food represents everything that is bad in their worlds. Most overeaters seldom taste more than the first bite or two of anything that they eat. The rest of the eating is punishment, because it is so involved with guilt and with anger.

You are about to develop a real appreciation for food. By not dividing your attention and by learning to enjoy your food, you will begin to develop a new way of thinking about the food that you eat. As you gain control of your eating behavior and you lose weight, food will no longer be a threat. Strict adherence to these easily managed tasks will automatically produce results. You will lose weight and also change unhealthy eating patterns. You will never be fat again.

Along with your focus on eating, the technique of eating as a separate activity will work, with eating only at appropriate places, to eliminate the external cues that trigger you to eat. For instance, the television commercial won't cue you to grab a snack. Or sitting in your favorite chair to read the newspaper won't automatically trigger you to think of food.

With this rule, a useful practice is never to talk with your fork in your hand. When you converse at the table, always put your fork down. Don't pick it up again until you finish talking and the conversation moves on to someone else. Remember, as a child, how many times you were told never to talk with your mouth full? Now is the time to recall rules that make you eat more thoughtfully and at a slower pace. Eat every meal as though you were dressed in formal clothing and dining at the White House with the President. Exaggerate for a while. Use all of the table manners that you can remember. Set the table carefully, especially for breakfast. Don't be self-conscious. Make every meal as elaborate and as pleasant as you can. Use special china and special eating utensils, and of course use cloth napkins. No guest can be more important than you are. No celebration is more deserving of a fine table setting than this reunion with yourself. Live it up! You have deprived yourself of beauty for the last time.

RULE 4

Use Thirty Minutes for Each Meal.
THIS IS THE MOST REWARDING RULE OF ALL, BUT may possibly be the most difficult one to master. Why? Because, almost without exception, fat people eat faster than anybody! If we had to identify any single factor most responsible for obesity, rapid eating would probably take the prize.

It takes about twenty minutes for your stomach to signal the behavior-control center in your brain that the stomach is full. In the Mannix Method we call the signal apparatus an "appestat." It functions like a thermostat for the appetite. If you watch babies and young children eating, you will discover that they stop eating rather abruptly when they are full. They respond immediately to the appestat signal. You did that too, when you were a child, and you stopped responding for some obscure reason. Perhaps you were forced to eat every morsel on your plate as a child, against your will. Whatever the causes are for your obesity, you can change the course of events now by responding to your appestat every time it signals. Give it time to signal (about twenty minutes), and react to the signal by not eating any more at that meal! Be reminded again that losing weight isn't like stopping a freight train. A thirty-minute requirement for each meal may bore you to tears for a while, but practice this task without fail for twenty-one days and it will become extremely comfortable. The majority of my clients even report that they look forward to taking thirty minutes to eat. It becomes a peaceful time of the day, and represents an easy way to control the environment.

Do not "occasionally" go back to your old habit of bolting

food, or eating in front of the refrigerator. You will be reinforcing old behavior at the same time that you are attempting to incorporate new behavior. You will undermine your success severely, leading to discouragement and possible failure. You have reinforced your poor eating habits thousands of times over the years. Each time you set yourself back to start again will diminish your confidence, and your self-esteem. Taking thirty minutes to eat every meal is time well invested for a handsome return. Enjoy your food.

Here are some directions for eating slowly and enjoying food more:

1. TAKE SMALL BITES. Small bites provide you with more eating activity and more taste sensation. With each bite of food your taste buds send messages to the appetite control center in your brain. The keener the sensation, the more active the control function becomes in registering satisfaction. The "stop" signal will signal sharply when your need for food has been met.

2. REPLACE YOUR FORK AFTER EACH BITE. Chew that bite thoroughly. Swallow and clear your mouth. Take a sip of water before you pick up your fork again to go back for another small bite. Small sips of water will help you pace your eating for the first week or so, and can be eliminated later. You are in training. Until your new eating techniques become automatic, it is helpful to overemphasize each task. Don't be fooled by the simplicity of these tasks. They are, indeed, simple, but they require your complete attention. So: Replace your fork after each bite, and chew your food carefully and well. In twenty-one days you will be able to depend on eating slowly. You will be in control.

3. TAKE TWO INTERMISSIONS. In your mind's eye divide each of your meals into three segments. About ten minutes after starting, push your chair away from the table. Adjust your sitting position. Take a deep breath. Hold that deep breath for the count of five and then exhale s-l-o-w-l-y. The air in your lungs will relax tension by lowering your heart rate and your blood pressure. This breathing tends to diminish the intensity of eating. Relax away from the table in this fashion for a minute or two. Then go back to taking small bites of food and replacing the fork between bites through each segment of the meal.

During the second intermission, it will be time for your appestat to signal that sufficient food has been consumed. Analyze your feeling. Stop eating if you are full. It takes some courage at first to fully accept the signal. You have been ignoring it for many years. If you feel satisfied enough to take you through to the next refueling time called a "meal," take the chance. Stop eating. You may have to leave a large amount of food on your plate. Try. The very worst thing that can happen is that you will be slightly hungrier for your next meal. Being a little hungry is far more comfortable than your usual feeling of being overstuffed. If you find at first that leaving food is too much for you to handle, use the "salting down trick." This trick is particularly handy in someone else's home, when leaving the table is not in order. That's right, you guessed correctly: Pour enough salt on the remaining food to make it awful! This will never be necessary after you learn control.

If, after an honest appraisal of your feeling of satisfaction, you still feel hungry, and the appestat agrees with you, by all means go back to your meal. But be prepared to be very sensitive to recognizing the stop signal after any bite, and be ready to stop immediately. Abandon your fork on your plate heaped with food, perhaps, the way you did when you were a child.

This new habit will be forever useful to you. Work at the technique until it is automatic, and you are master. It requires patience, but you will be grateful. You will be grateful for a healthy lifetime.

YOUR WEIGHT LOSS RECORD

Your weight loss will serve only as an indicator of how successful you are at learning *control.* You have lost weight before—many times perhaps. So in isolation, the loss of weight means nothing. The objective of the Mannix Method is to help you to develop *control* resulting in weight loss and to master *control* for continuous good management after you have lost body fat. Therefore, realize that the daily loss of weight is the consequence of *control* and not your ultimate reward. The successful incorporation of good eating habits, and the ease with which you make these habits part of your everyday behavior, are the true, ultimate rewards. Loss of weight is automatic when your food intake satisfies the body needs for fuel, and not your emotional need for gorging.

YOUR WEIGHT GRAPH

The weight graph in the back of the book is for recording your weight changes. Please weigh yourself *once a week only*. Record your weight on the graph with a dot in the proper square above the date. Connect the dots with a line each week and continue this procedure throughout the program as shown. The connected

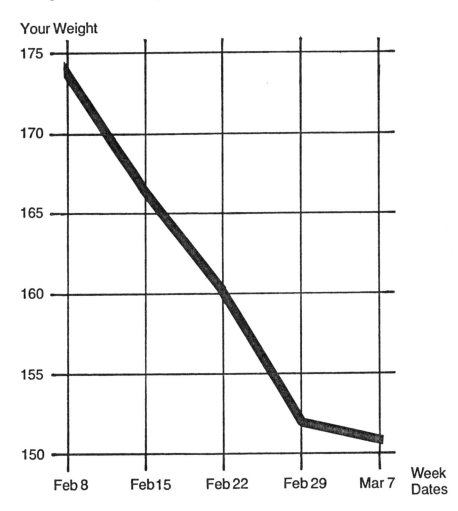

Your Weight

lines will show you the trend of weight change, and will indicate your degree of success. Do not weigh yourself more than once a week. Deny yourself the temptation. Establish one day of the week for weighing yourself. Weigh in before breakfast. Record your weight on the graph and then hide the scale until the next week at the same time. You don't need the scale to tell you if you feel heavy or light. The actual number equivalent of that feeling means very little. The emphasis in the Mannix Method is on control and on success. Weigh yourself only once a week, and use that information only for graphing change as the result of your new behavior. Begin to think and act like the liberated person you can be, involved in living, unhampered by an obsession with weight.

SUMMARY

Success breeds success. Your successful completion of Session 1 will lay a firm foundation for the success of the whole program. Understand all techniques in each session before beginning each session. Follow the directions precisely. Commit yourself to each session for the week and practice every technique thoroughly. Dedicate yourself to one week at a time. Dedicate yourself to one session at a time, to feeling comfortable with your commitment. You will appreciate weekly results enough to move you on to the next session.

Be flexible! Be receptive to improvement. Change sometimes threatens one's security, but as Franklin Delano Roosevelt said, "The only thing we have to fear is fear itself." Face your need and do something about it. You feel trapped. This is an easy way to freedom.

Weigh yourself the first morning and mark your weight on the graph. Practice each task with understanding and purpose, and repeat the method through each session.

On the contract that follows, sign your initials on the line provided, to designate your commitment to yourself, for Session 1. Pledge your best to get your best!

Commit yourself by signing the following contract.

Remember that this is a point of honor—a private obligation to yourself:

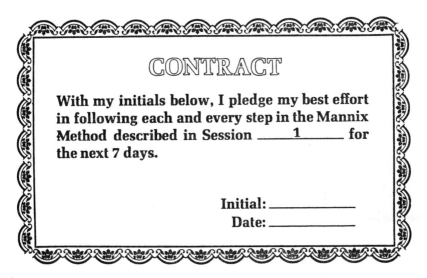

HIGHLIGHTS

A. Tapered Eating

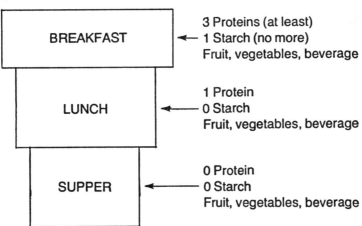

No food for at least four hours before retiring.

Include vegetables, fruit, and beverages with an eye to calories.

B. Behavior Rules

1. Record everything that you eat in your Journal *before* you eat it.
2. Eat only at an appropriate eating place.
3. Eat only. Perform no other activity when you eat.
4. Take thirty minutes for each meal.
5. Use appestat control. Respond to signals.

C. Twenty-one Days to Build a Habit

Repeat each task for twenty-one days with proper attitudes. REINFORCEMENT makes behavior dependable.

D. Weight Chart

1. Weigh yourself only once a week, at the same time of day.
2. Record your weight on the graph in the appendix at the end of this book.
3. Connect the weight marks on the chart to plot your progress in changing your behavior.

E. Time for Session 1

1. In the Mannix Method Session 1 is practiced for seven days.
2. Begin Session 2 on the eighth day.

SESSION 2

FEEL GOOD

In my clinic I meet with clients at least once a week. In reviewing their progress, I find that each person has different strengths and weaknesses in working through the skills introduced in Session 1. Each person is different in his/her approach and in his/her commitment, but everyone seems to experience a good feeling of accomplishment—despite some possibly mediocre performance some of the time.

You are probably feeling better than you have felt for ages. It is not unusual to hear clients report that they sleep better, have more energy, and have lost old compulsive urges for particular foods. If you share those experiences, you are beginning to enjoy rewards and are on your way to changing previous failure to future success.

Now that you feel healthier, be reminded that good health is one of the most prized possessions in life. Your eating had become an obsessive hobby, but because you are controlling your eating patterns and feeling better because of that control, it is time now to analyze the pleasure you always thought you derived from food. The real pleasure from food comes from the feeling of well-being that food provides, not from a fleeting taste sensation.

You have only just begun to tap the benefits derived from educated eating. Feel positive and good about the progress that you have made, and use your momentum to try a little harder this week. Follow procedures meticulously. Changing old familiar behavior takes practice and determination.

In one short week you recognize improvement. It's quite easy. You are doing something about a condition that has been haunting you, and you are succeeding. Go into this second session with the strength of a winner. Your weight graph most likely charts a loss—that is, if you kept the bargain that you made with yourself to use every technique learned in Session 1. The weight graph is a good way to mark progress. However, there is the possibility that you followed your eating outline perfectly all week and show no weight loss. People differ. People metabolize foods differently. This is one of the reasons for emphasizing that the goal in the Mannix Method of weight control is to change the behavior that leads to excess weight. Weight loss will be inevitable.

If you did show a weight loss this first week, do not become complacent and assume that you are in control. That kind of reasoning may result in a slow but certain return to old established behavior. You will then slip back to where you started, with an even greater feeling of defeat. Increase your effort now. You have actually been through the most difficult session of all. Your adventure becomes more interesting and exciting as you go on.

THROW YOUR WEIGHT AROUND

Now let's talk about your ability to assert yourself. Being assertive at this stage in your training is extremely useful. The environment keeps fat people fat. Your family, advertising, quick foods, junk foods, and your defeatist attitude all help to perpetuate your fat. It can get worse before it gets better, so you must develop the ability to detach yourself from the destructive forces in your surroundings.

An enormous food industry has grown more concerned with transportation, profit, and promotion than with quality. They will package and sell anything that you will buy. Huge conglomerates market the food you eat with profit as their primary motive. The artificial additives in our foods may contribute to cancer and to other diseases. We are lured into eating junk foods that poison our systems. Extra salt on peanuts and chips makes you eat more and more and more. Clever advertising challenges you to try to eat only one, implying that the product is so delicious that you can't stop eating it. The truth is that it is usually greasy and salty, very salty, and you taste nothing but the salt. You keep eating without thought, like a puppet on a string, in an automatic way. Similarly, sugar in candy, cakes, cookies, and pastries is addictive. You never feel satisfied, so you eat more and more and more. Americans eat more than 150 pounds of sugar per person each year. An insignificant amount of that sugar comes directly from the sugar bowl; the rest is in hidden places. The next time you are in a market, read some of the labels on the foods that you select. Choose any item at random. Chances are that you will find sugar listed as one of the first ingredients. (Ingredients on labels are listed by their volume.) There is sugar in canned vegetables, condiments, sauces, cereals, breads, peanut butter, soups etc. . . . Almost every packaged food contains sugar. If you really want to explore, find the huge breakfast cereal aisle in a supermarket and try to find a package of cereal that contains no sugar. You may find two in a possible dozen. How about ice cream? The manufacturers of ice cream are not required by law to list the ingredients in their product. Consequently most ice creams are largely synthetic. Eggs have been replaced by an emulsifier borrowed from the chemical petroleum industry. Flavorings are practically all imitation and are petroleum based. The concoction is colored with dye to resemble the flavor. It is too late to hope to reform the food industry. It may even become worse. It is, therefore, your responsibility to insist on better foods. You must affect your own environment to affect your eating. Don't be the fool anymore!

There are just four inches from your mouth to your swallow. You are fat because of that short distance, which represents a rather short thrill. You distort your body and your personality and destroy so many nice things in your life for that short distance of taste excitement. With that in mind, begin this session with a stronger commitment. You can control your life. You have already started. The biggest step, the giant step, was your first step.

FOOD JOURNAL

A Food Journal is a written record of all the food that you eat each day.

Everyone, after keeping the Food Journal for the first week, can find areas for improvement. It will be the exceptional individual who keeps the perfect Journal at first try. If you are that exceptional person, this program will be particularly easy. You can bank on building new and appropriate eating behavior rapidly and permanently in a very short time.

The most common pitfall in keeping a Food Journal is neglect. You must record what you eat just *before* you eat it. Write before you eat! The purpose is to think before you leap—to borrow a phrase. The purpose in writing before you eat is to put you in control of choosing what you eat, and perhaps deciding *if* you want to eat it. Writing before you eat allows you to plan and to anticipate eating, which you rarely did until you were introduced to the Mannix Method. Your old patterns of eating encouraged confession rather than intelligent anticipation. Remember when you found yourself finishing a piece of cake or candy before you realized that you had eaten it? There is no longer room for that kind of irresponsible, "forgetful" eating. You are now the Captain, not the Culprit. Put an end to the whole unhappy scene immediately by *writing what you eat before you eat it!* The rewards are enormous. The Food Journal is a temporary tool, so for the short few weeks that you use it, reap its benefits. *Write before you eat.*

The next most common pitfall in keeping the Food Journal is the inaccurate recording of your "eating time." It is important to record the exact amount of time that it took you to eat. It was probably awkward for you to use thirty minutes to eat each of your meals. This week, however, you will be more comfortable. Make it a practice to go back to your Journal after you have finished eating and to record the exact amount of time it took you to complete your meal. If your eating time was less than thirty minutes, it may be assumed that you left food on your plate.

Make a note of that in your Journal along with your "eating time." With this technique, you learn to respond to your appestat, the signal that tells you that you have filled your stomach with enough food to satisfy your needs. Without this clever signal sounding loud and clear, you have to guess at the amount of fuel you need—and that guessing has proved to be very unreliable in the past.

A client of mine who has just completed the first week on Tapered Eating protested, before starting the Mannix Method, that he was a serious meat eater and didn't care for salads or for vegetables. He ate only meat and usually huge quantities of it at one time. Today he registered a six-pound weight loss and boasted of a perfect Food Journal, with the exception of one Saturday-night meal. That meal was at his wife's birthday dinner in a restaurant where he could not order a salad. He chose fish instead of his usual choice of meat, in an attempt to keep as close to his schedule as was possible. He was very proud of his control and was excited about the results. He reported feeling tremendously lighter (his actual weight was 296 pounds), sleeping better, and having no desire for food after dinner, which had usually been the case in the evening. He even reported that he was never depressed at any time throughout the whole week.

The Food Journal is a written feedback on your stumbling blocks and on your progress. It gives you very important feedback. Write everything that you eat in the Journal *before* you eat it. It is the only way you will benefit from the Food Journal.

CUE ELIMINATION

All of us are stimulated to eat at various times by cues coming from the environment. Ideally, hunger should be the only cue to eat, but very often the sight of food, or odors, or just watching someone else eat, cues us to want to eat. The elimination of the simple and more obvious cues from the environment can be achieved by practicing two behavior skills. Memorize what they are:

1. Eat only at designated eating places.
2. Perform no other activity while you eat.

The environment helps to keep fat people fat. In order to have that environment serve you rather than hinder you, you must assert yourself about food and about eating. Some of the techniques you will practice to eliminate environmental cueing may require that you ask for the cooperation of the other members of your household. Assert yourself—which really means speak up, don't take a backseat. Ask the other members of your household for a helping hand. Most family members will try to cooperate in removing some obstacles for you. Keep in mind, however, that they have watched you perform "diet" regimes before and they don't have much faith in your success with losing weight. They have heard your song before. So be patient with their impatience. As they see you succeeding with the Mannix Method of behavior modification, you will probably find them examining this manual now and again to learn some of your techniques. Most clients report that after a few weeks, family members— spouses and children—want to adopt Tapered Eating. Life around the house then becomes more manageable. At first, however, verbalize your needs. Assert yourself, but be patient. Tell the members of your family about your plan, assume that they will give assistance with the least amount of resistance, and give them time to change.

The last page of this session is a graph for you to diagram a floor plan of your living quarters. Then:

1. Mark an X at all the places where you have been accustomed to eating.
2. Circle all X's that are not proper eating places.
3. Next, go through your house, and on the floor plan mark F at all of the places where you can now find food. Be especially careful to examine the places where you already have a circled X.
4. Now, with diagram in hand, check back to all the non-kitchen places marked with an F. Remove all of the food that you find there. Put it in the kitchen.
5. Circle the F to indicate that the food has been removed.

From that diagram, you can now see by the circled X's and circled F's where some dangerous environmental cues are hidden. You have already eliminated eating at taboo places by storing your food in the kitchen. Last week's session eliminated eating at undesignated places by giving you the behavior rule of eating only at an appropriate eating place. It is now time to eliminate those cues completely.

A sample floor plan is shown:

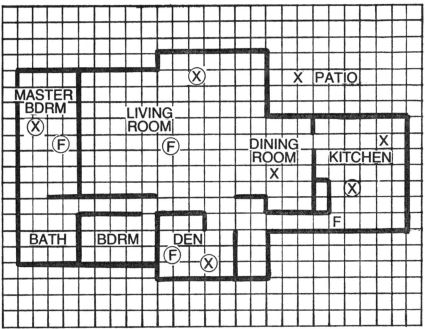

Sample Floor Plan

Go back to all the circled X's—places that are not proper eating places—and change at least one aspect of the activity that you perform at that place. For instance, if you find a circled X in the television room, go to that room and change something about your ritual of watching television. Make the change obviously different. Perhaps you can rearrange your chairs. Or switch places on the couch with others in the family. Try rearranging the room completely. Make everything about the activity different. Consider moving the television set to another room for a few weeks. Do you see the point? Changing patterns is the idea! Change some part of every one of your activities in any place of your living space shown on your diagram as a place of eating, or a place where food is stored. It may take a little ingenuity, but the change doesn't have to be monumental. Just make noticeable changes. Those changes will be enough to remind you that something is different about your activity, and that reminder will be enough to help you to eliminate cues to eat. These changes may seem clumsy for a while, but stick with them. They will become comfortable, and with that feeling of comfort you will develop control. You will control eating cues and eating times. In fact, you will be in control of anything you want to do with you.

COST RESPONSE

You have now removed all available foods to the kitchen. Understanding "cost response" may be useful at this point. The cost-response principle is based on the fact that overeaters, as a rule, will not go to any trouble to prepare their snacks. They generally use the least possible amount of energy and effort to get food. They will eat almost anything and they are devoted to precooked foods and to preparations. Their expenditure of energy is usually minimal. Their response is lazy. In other words, their response costs very little effort. With that information, it is a very good idea to change the storage spots in your kitchen. Assign all cookies and other high-calorie snacks to inconvenient areas. These snacks are presumably kept for other family members. A high cupboard shelf that is out of normal reach is the best place. Put all the cookies, candies, nuts, crackers, breads, etc., in one of these out-of-the-way places. Tell other family members where all the "junk foods" are stored and ask them to replace packages in the assigned area after helping themselves. Be assertive and let them know that you are prepared to discard any snack food that is left carelessly around the house or even in the kitchen. And do just that if you have to! I have one client who prepared a food-storage cabinet in the garage and assigned all snack foods to that cabinet. The energy expenditure of going out of the kitchen, through the laundry room, down the stairs, and into the garage kept her from eating the food. It also discouraged the rest of her family from taking the trouble to snack. Eventually all the garage food was thrown away and snack foods were completely eliminated in her house.

Serve all meals from the kitchen. Do not use serving plates at the table. Change family-style serving. This may be a real departure from your usual mealtime procedure, and may be altered later. However, at this point in your control it is important to serve from the kitchen, with portions of food placed directly on plates. As you are developing techniques for responding to your appestat signal, it makes good sense to minimize pitfalls. This again uses the cost-response principle. If food is not readily available on the table, you may not be inclined to exert the effort to get second portions after you know that you have had enough to eat. So serve each meal from the kitchen and prepare just enough to be eaten at that one meal. If you do have some food to be stored after a meal, cover the food to be stored immediately and be swift about discarding all the scraps. Don't eat that small slice of meat on Tommy's plate because you hate to waste. Throw it away! Waste it! Don't waist it!

OUT OF SIGHT

The next cue elimination will be to cover the food in the refrigerator. Use foil or opaque containers. Remember, if you can't see the food, it will minimize its attraction. Another one of my clients told me of a very useful technique: She would wrap all food and leftovers in aluminum foil and then use a piece of masking tape on the top to write a description of the contents. When it was time to prepare meals, she could easily select the food that she would be cooking just by reading the labels. This method caused little complaint from her family, and it eliminated the visual cue of seeing food whenever she opened the refrigerator. Remove visual cues wherever possible!

After you have finished your chores in the kitchen, leave the kitchen with no intention of returning again until you are hungry for your next meal. Try putting a sign on the kitchen door that says "closed until breakfast."

Another useful technique is to shop for food only when you are not hungry. Never, never shop on an empty stomach. Think of the money you will save! You will be amazed at your ability to resist junk if you have just had a full meal. Exercising control will be easy.

You have systematically eliminated cues and have reduced your exposure to food. In reducing your exposure to food, you will find it possible to gauge the proper times to eat. Don't ever permit yourself to be hungry, but remember, too—do not even eat unless you *are* hungry! With the limited availability of food, and with the honest use of your Food Journal and learned behavior rules, you are now equipped to plan what you will eat. You will eat with discrimination and control. You are changing eating patterns rapidly. Hold to your course! Be enthusiastic; don't resist your body's natural tendency to improve and to seek a healthier condition.

IF YOU EAT, MAKE IT WORTHWHILE

Anyone who has abused food to become overweight doesn't really enjoy food. It is now time to develop pleasure in eating. Foods create feelings. If you are using thirty minutes for each of your meals, you must be experiencing taste sensations that you never knew before. Explore those food messages. Close your eyes and chew each "new" food slowly twenty-five times. Then feel, really feel, the food slide down your throat. How does it taste? What does the texture feel like? How long does the taste last? Does the taste change as you chew? Experience the food that you are eating.

You may find that some of the foods you think you love best are eliminated simply with this method of analysis—of experiencing each mouthful of food. Along with the analysis of your problem foods, compare, with the same method, some of the foods that are considered "good" foods, such as fruits and vegetables. The revelation may astound you. Your "problem" foods may lose a good deal of their appeal. The healthful foods, in contrast, may delight you. Then work on enjoying good food when your energy demands the most fuel, and then taper the amount as your day comes to an end.

Decorate your tables at home with care and with an eye for beauty. This was mentioned before, but should be stressed again. Use your best dinner china, napkins, and silver. Set an elaborate table and include a candle—even at breakfast time if it is dark outside. Make eating a pleasurable time. It is one of the delights of the world. Enjoy it! Eat gourmet style. Never mix foods in the same bite. Always take the time to chew thoroughly. Take the time to taste. Sip a beverage in between bites of different foods to freshen your mouth for the next taste treat. Take your time to relax. You are using thirty minutes to eat; use them with pleasure. Enjoy food! Remember, it is not food that is your problem, but the way you eat that food.

MAKE IT A MEAL

If you are hungry and are going to permit yourself to eat in between your meals or after your dinner, make that food another meal, complete with all the rules and procedures you follow at all of your meals. The most important element when allowing yourself extra food is to eliminate the panic of eating and the guilt that follows. You can systematically eliminate panic, and perhaps the extra food, completely. Write what you are about to eat in your Food Journal. Then arrange the food on a special plate. If the snack is something like a fruit, cut it up into small pieces and arrange it on the plate. Whatever the food is, determine your portion and take it to a designated eating place. Relax and enjoy the food by taking small bites. Taste your tempting treat. If you are going to eat it, make it worth your while!

Of course, you are working to eliminate any between-meal eating, but while your sense of commitment and responsibility is developing and growing, at least eliminate panic snacking and compulsive stuffing by treating everything that you eat with the importance of a meal. Eat as a gourmet does, with deliberation, a keen sense of taste, and appreciation.

SUMMARY

Begin this second session with a complete review and evaluation of last week's Food Journal. Use extra effort to make your Food Journal more perfect this week.

The Food Journal is important as the major source of feedback for you, so that you may follow your progress in gaining control. The Food Journal is also a valuable planning guide to help you to anticipate control. It will be discontinued in the ninth week, so use it conscientiously for this relatively short time. Keep it with you all the time, and write in it before you eat anything. Write before you eat!

Always keep in mind that it takes twenty-one days to establish a habit. Expend your effort now. These next three weeks will build the groundwork for the continued control of the food in your life. Every time you reinforce your old established eating habits, you set yourself back. So practice your new behaviors to the letter; be patient. It's really very very easy.

Continue practicing all behavior rules from Session 1:

1. Write before you eat.
2. Eat at appropriate eating places only.
3. Eat only—perform no other activity when you eat.
4. Take thirty minutes for each meal:

take small bites;
replace your fork between bites;
take two intermissions during each meal.

Never perform any other activity while you are eating. Don't break this rule. One of my clients casually mentioned to me, after a few weeks on the Method, that she was observing every one of the behavior rules "to the letter." Except, of course, she watched a morning show on television while she ate her breakfast. Watching the show was such an established ritual that she didn't consider it an activity. After she discontinued that practice, she discovered she was more easily able to eliminate her midmorning snack, and more successful in spending thirty minutes on each of her meals. She began to assume a more aggressive attitude about her work on the Mannix Method. Just that one oversight of watching television during breakfast disrupted her practice schedule . . . to her detriment. It retarded her weight loss.

Before you begin this week's session, review your Food Journal. Make sure that you are aware of reading the newspaper, writing lists of errands, listening to the news on the radio, or watching television. If you find one or two times with "double activities," circle them in your Journal and be prepared to alter the circumstance the next time around. If your family watches a morning show on television, change your place of eating to the dining room. Or change the location of the television set so that you may eat without being disturbed. Assert yourself. Your life depends on it. Establish your rights.

Tapered Eating should be continued through this week with no deviation. Build strong behavior patterns so that this tapered style becomes your preferred way of eating. Once you have done that, you will be able to be more flexible. After you have re-shaped your behavior and your body, you may add some protein to your dinners occasionally, or you may have a sandwich for lunch every once in a while. Chances are that you won't want to indulge. You will have adopted this new way of life. Your old patterns will prove uncomfortable and unsatisfying to you. For the moment, however, practice the energy-demand style and use all learned behavior rules. You will have more energy and will sleep restfully. Those rewards will help you increase momentum and commit yourself with determination. The first two sessions are the most demanding. Start this second week with confidence and purpose, building on last week's success and useful new be-havior patterns.

Commit yourself by signing the following contract.

Remember that this is a point of honor—a private obligation to yourself:

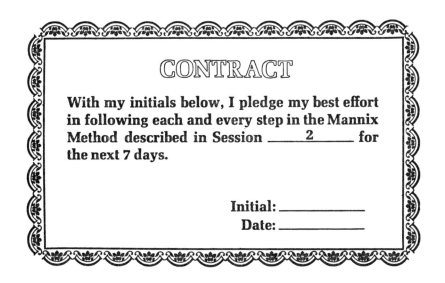

CONTRACT

With my initials below, I pledge my best effort in following each and every step in the Mannix Method described in Session ____2____ for the next 7 days.

Initial: _____

Date: _____

HIGHLIGHTS

A. Review Your Food Journal

1. Check for thirty minutes for each meal (rate).
2. Write before you eat.
3. Record every morsel that you eat. Include all beverages except water.
4. Keep legible records. Sloppy records will result in sloppy eating practices.
5. Finish all food four hours before you retire.

B. Cue Elimination

1. Remove food to the kitchen from every other room.
2. Use your house diagram to change one aspect of every activity that has up to now included food (for example television in the den, reading in bed, ironing in laundry room).
3. Change your place at the dinner table.
4. Remove all snacks in the kitchen to unused storage space.
5. Serve all meals from the kitchen, not at the table family style.
6. Shop for food after you have eaten, on a full stomach.
7. Always use a list. Never do impulse shopping.

C. If You Eat It, Make It Important

1. No sneak eating.
2. No guilt-producing eating. Guilt is as destructive as improper eating.
3. Enjoy your food. Make it worth your while.
4. Set pretty tables.
5. Take small bites.

D. Eat Meals—Eat No Snacks

Apply all behavior rules whenever and whatever you eat.

E. Weight Chart

1. Weigh yourself only once each week.
2. Graph your weekly weight on the chart.
3. Make this an incidental activity. A scale is not a home.

F. Time Allotment

1. Session 2, like Session 1, takes one whole week to complete.
2. Begin Session 3 on the eighth day.

FLOOR PLAN OF MY LIVING SPACE

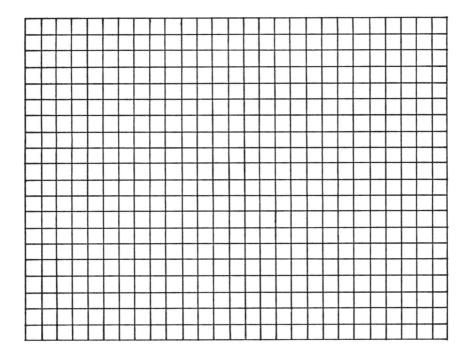

SESSION 3

INTERMITTENT REINFORCEMENT

You are now starting a very important week with the Mannix Method. The third week will complete the twenty-one days necessary for establishing a "habit." Your new eating patterns can be considered dependable at this point in their development. You have been involved in the Mannix Method for the past two weeks, and you can see and recognize changes in your attitude about food. You are comfortable and secure with relaxed but deliberate eating. You are well on the way to mastering permanent control of your eating. This is the path to your goals. Stick to your course and be very careful now to practice every technique with meticulous care. Make no changes. Add nothing. Omit nothing.

The most rapid and the most thorough way to disrupt your progress and possibly eliminate your chances for success is with *intermittent reinforcement.* Intermittent reinforcement is the process by which behavior is rewarded at irregular intervals. It reinforces the strongest kind of devotion to that behavior. In the context of your behavior training, this refers to your occasional "cheating," to your relaxation of behavior rules, and to those small deviations from the Tapered style of your meals.

The most effective way to build subconscious dedication to anything—a person, a job, a habit, or even a small pleasure—is to enjoy its reward irregularly: every now and then. The exact same reward experienced all of the time would make you less dependent on that particular behavior. With intermittent reinforcement you must divorce or separate yourself many times. With each separation, the chances of returning become greater.

The most dramatic example of intermittent reinforcement is demonstrated in Las Vegas at the gambling tables. The only thing that attracts the gambler to the game is the chance of winning occasionally. If he were rewarded all of the time for each of his efforts, it would become the same old thing and he would become disenchanted. Occasional success makes him feel triumphant if he can leave the game with no loss or perhaps a small loss, anticipating the occasional "win."

Slot machine devotees are an obvious example of that kind of rewarded behavior. The addicted slot-machine player will feed the machine extravagantly, anticipating the inevitable but occasional payoff. He watches the machine that he is playing while he canvasses the area to see if any other player gives up after depositing large amounts of money without waiting for the return. If he should spot a well-fed abandoned machine, he may switch machines in the hope that the other machine is closer to the payoff. Such people are motivated by the dynamics of intermittent reinforcement—the periodic or irregular return on the investment. Their dedication is reinforced by the occasional small return with the clamor of bells and flashing lights that signal the "win." All they need is to see or to hear about a big winner, to keep them driven toward the goal.

Intermittent reinforcement builds obsession. Obsession reinforces dependence.

If you fall prey to intermittent reinforcement—let's say by eating in front of the television set—you will never extinguish the influence of television on your desire to eat. You will be so receptive to the television cue, you will develop a fear of eating each time you watch television. You will be triggered to eat or you will be triggered to resist your urge to eat. In either case, you will associate eating with watching television.

Think of other examples of intermittent reinforcement and its subsequent enslavement. Did you ever separate from a loved one? The easiest way to get over that kind of separation is to change your life-style to eliminate the things that you shared. Remove the reminders. What a mistake it is to keep old photographs and souvenirs, or to see his or her car parked around town, or to sit at the same familiar table in your favorite restaurant. That kind of intermittent reminder of someone you want to forget will keep you emotionally involved forever. The best way to gain independence, emotional independence, is to move away. Change your total environment. Eliminate the reminders. The complete break is necessary at some point. Occasional involvement is complicated and difficult.

How about the alcoholic? Before an alcoholic reforms, he usually tries many ways of cutting down on his drinking. He may even stop drinking completely for a week or for a month without great difficulty. Each time he goes back for that first drink, he is casual and has no real need. But that first drink brings a torrent of binge drinking that becomes worse with each new start. He is reinforcing his habit intermittently. He is building an obsession that will lead to the most hopeless addiction. Abstaining from drinking totally is much easier for the person with a drinking problem than the stopping over and over again. Continuous reinforcement, all or nothing at all—one hundred percent on or one hundred percent off—provides the best chance for recovery and for permanent control.

Cigarette smoking is another good example of the possible dangers of intermittent reinforcement. A cigarette smoker is addicted to the substance nicotine and to the activity (behavior) of smoking. He has a physical need for nicotine, and a psychological need for the smoking ritual. The easiest way to break the habit of smoking is to stop smoking completely. One must allow the body to detoxify, to alter the need for those chemicals, and to develop alternate patterns of behavior to replace smoking behavior. Both steps are necessary to train a person to be a nonsmoker. One part without the other will nourish the need and the desire to smoke. A return to nicotine is guaranteed.

Intermittent reinforcement of any behavior creates the strongest addiction. The best way to develop new patterns of behavior is to reinforce the new behavior exclusively—one hundred percent. Do not return to old patterns of behavior occasionally until dependable new habits have replaced them and are providing more satisfying rewards than did the old ones. With the gambler, the alcoholic, and the smoker, the effects of occasional reinforcement are dramatically observable. With a person controlling weight, the damage done by intermittent reinforcement is insidious and slow. You may still lose weight, but you will not be released from your addiction to eating. You will gain your weight again. You will gain every pound that you struggle to lose.

Do not ever reinforce your old eating behavior while you are at work on the Mannix Method of control. During Session 8 you are permitted to relax this restriction. So stay meticulously dedicated until the time is right to be more flexible. With no intermittent reinforcement of old behavior patterns, you will develop new habits and new attitudes that will change your entire approach to eating. Allow those actions and attitudes the time to develop. Allow yourself to change so that you may be free from addiction.

One word of caution. Be very careful not to modify the program at this time. Many of us think that we are ready to solo long before our actual ability is sufficient to handle the challenge. Your success with the Mannix Method will enhance every facet of your living. Follow each session to the letter for exactly the specified time. At the end of this session you will have completed your basic twenty-one-day time goal. You will then begin to refine and to detail your new eating habits. Your old negative patterns will be replaced. Your reward will be worthy of your investment.

TOTAL BEHAVIOR AND HABIT ANALYSIS

You are changing a behavior that has had an unbelievably prominent spot in your life. Eating is part of so many of your activities and your moods. It has been your reward for achievement and your solace for disappointment. Until you started the Mannix Method, food seemed to be part of everything. You have started to alter that, and are now ready to really separate eating from all of the other things that you do. You may now examine its real function.

To examine any one function that is enmeshed with many other functions, it must be isolated or separated. It must be "singled."

Try to alter one single part of each of your rituals every day this week. Start in the morning and change one (or more if you feel adventurous) link in the chain of your morning "getting-ready" ritual. We all have a preferred ritual of preparation in the morning. Change some single part of your usual morning ritual. If you usually arise and go directly to the kitchen to start the coffee or to prepare breakfast, take your shower first and then get dressed before starting the coffee. Rearrange one of your activities. Or go back to bed to read the paper instead of reading it at your usual spot. Then resume your other preparation activities. Change one single thing in the first ritual of your day, then change one small sequence in every other daily ritual. You actually have dozens of these familiar patterns of behavior that require no thinking. They are automatic. Try sleeping on the other side of your bed. Getting out of bed on the opposite side would be one change in your morning ritual. Try putting a load of clothes in your washing machine as soon as you arise, or go out for a short walk. To start your day, consider washing your car, or writing a letter or reading a chapter of a good book. Rearrange some single part of your starting ritual, no matter how small the change may seem.

As your day progresses, alter something about every habit pattern that you can identify. After your morning ritual, take a slightly different route to work, or park in a different space. Brush your dog in the morning instead of brushing him in the afternoon. Use the afternoon to go to the park to watch children play. Make a list of your day's activities, then list small changes that you can make in each of those activities. The more changes you can make in your daily habit patterns, the easier it will be to change those that are not working for you and to identify your eating patterns.

The idea is to change behavior patterns, not particular activities. It would be pointless, for example, to write with your "other hand" or to wear socks of a different color. You want to identify "patterns" of behavior. Leave the house in the morning by the back door, rearrange the sequence of your housecleaning, change the location of your desk and telephone at work. Use the elevator for part of the way and walk the rest. Take a walk at lunch, plan a bath when you return home, back your car into the garage, or exchange your parking spot with your spouse or neighbor. There are countless changes that you can make during your day, if you look for them. Any small change in every identifiable ritual will help you to understand the place eating has in your activities.

You will undoubtedly discover at least one ritual that no longer works for you. We all have a tendency to hold on to the things that once provided pleasure. We hold on long after circumstances have changed their usefulness. Be prepared to face some things that may seem functional but in reality are obsolete. They may be as harmful as your eating rituals have become. You are now making changes in your life. Examine everything at the same time and rearrange your life to serve you better, if you can. You know you perform one ritual that doesn't serve you well— your eating ritual. It seems entirely possible that there are others. Begin today to examine the rituals that comprise your life. Evaluate those rituals that no longer serve you well.

Join the spirit of total behavior and habit analysis. Search out all of your little daily behavior chains and change some one thing in each chain. It can be fun. Contemplating change may frighten, but once started, change can be exciting, revitalizing, and very easy. It is important for you to begin. The time is now! The time is right!

When I was a child, my family went to the seashore for the summer. My mother taught me how to go into the ocean through the breaking waves. She taught me to run full speed into the surf, diving into an approaching wave. Other bathers walked into the waves and turned their backs to the surf. The breaking waves battered and tossed them about. By understanding the surf and then moving at full speed, at the right time, my mother showed me how to avoid being tossed and pained by getting wet. Try that now. Choose your time to move with habit analysis, and then run into the surf. Many overweight people tend to be savers and collectors. They are uncomfortable with the idea of change. If you are a saver, a protector of the status quo, risk some change now. Risk some security to find a better way. Take a deep breath and plunge into this technique with courage. Be reminded, once again, that the only thing we have to fear is fear itself.

Don't fool yourself with bluffing habit changes that leave you just as trapped in your old rituals as ever. Keep in mind that you may be uncomfortable with just the idea of change. Guard against being lazy and uninvolved. Make real changes. Borrow some energy from your original commitment. Do not ·permit yourself less than your very best effort. Dive in to swim.

FOOD JOURNAL

Your Food Journal is now giving you some positive feedback. Notice that your pace is more consistent. Your Attitude indicates that you are more relaxed when you eat. Look back through the pages to appreciate your progress. Check to see that you are still eating at least three proteins for breakfast, one protein and no starch for lunch, and no protein and no starch for supper. Do you know that avocado is a protein? So if you are including it in your salads at night it should be eliminated. Beans, corn, and peas are in the starch category. Watch for them in your Journal.

Be accurate with your Journal. Make very sure that you *write before you eat.*

The Journal serves much of its function as you write down all the food that you eat *before* you eat it. At the end of each week, review your Journal. First, look for obvious deviations from the Tapered, energy-demand style of eating. Then check the pace of each meal and the intermissions. There is never any reason to be hungry with the Mannix Method of eating. Check the amount of time in between your meals. If your breakfast is at 7 A.M. and you lunch at 2 P.M. you are waiting too long between those two meals for food, and you should be concerned that your blood sugar may drop. This may result in a real threat at suppertime or after supper, and lead to snacking between 9 P.M. and 11 P.M.

If you are hungry during the day or after your supper, look back through your Journal to see if your first two meals were sufficient and were spaced properly. Do not ever adjust the Mannix Method by introducing your own favorite little diet tricks to rush things along. Follow this Method exactly, word for word and to the letter. DO NOT DIET! You must eat to lose weight. You must eat to develop the kind of eating habits that allow you to be rid of the nagging "fattening food" clamor. Use your Journal to look for trends. Watch for old habits taking their place. The Journal tells you about your progress in changing old, destructive eating habits. Weight loss, prized indeed, is not necessarily an indicator of behavior change. So don't judge your success by weight loss alone. Keep a critical eye on your Journal. Don't allow yourself any room for a less-than-perfect record of your healthy eating behavior. The Journal tells you where you stand at any given moment.

Keep your Journal with accuracy. *Write before you eat. Review* the Journal each week before starting a new session. *Relax* and *pace* your meals for thirty minutes. You are your own therapist with this Method. Be objective with your review and your evaluation. You have everything to lose so that you may win! Stand by your commitment!

SUMMARY

Session 3 is an important week for you. You will complete the twenty-one-day period to establish new behavior. Be meticulous now! It is human nature to take liberties at the first sign of success, feeling that you have become the master. Instead, try a little harder. Don't stop progress with this little bit of self-deception. You have been fat too long to believe an easy solution in such a short time. You will work at this for twelve weeks. Not a day less. Stick with it. Don't free-lance and pick and choose the techniques that you think are important and disregard others. The Mannix Method is designed for you to lose your excess weight and to permanently change the behavior that causes you to gain weight—a-gain and a-gain. Every day will bring you closer to your goal. You will succeed! My clients have lost tons of weight.

Your major job for this session is to identify and to change the order of as many behavior patterns as you can. This exercise will help to make your eating behavior changes much easier. It is a simple technique, but like all of the other techniques, it requires some time and some precision. Appreciate the contribution that this session will make to your ability to be flexible and to feel secure with change. Change is one of the absolute certainties in your life. Face it, prepared to enjoy every moment.

Commit yourself by signing the following contract.
Remember that this is a point of honor—a private obligation to yourself:

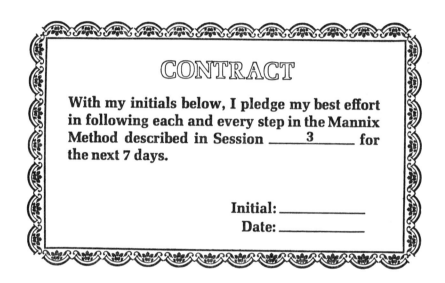

CONTRACT

With my initials below, I pledge my best effort in following each and every step in the Mannix Method described in Session ____3____ for the next 7 days.

Initial: _____
Date: _____

HIGHLIGHTS

A. Reinforcement

1. Intermittent reinforcement is the occasional reinforcement of old habits.
2. Intermittent reinforcement builds the strongest addiction.
3. Intermittent reinforcement eliminates the possibility of establishing new, dependable patterns of behavior.
4. Continuous reinforcement (one hundred percent on or one hundred percent off) allows behavior to change with the least resistance.
5. Continuous reinforcement of your new eating patterns for twenty-one days will establish your new behavior.

B. *Total Behavior and Habit Analysis*

1. Examine any part of a chain of behavior by separating it. "Single" it.
2. Change one link in every identifiable behavior chain every day this week.
3. Change parts of behavior patterns, not individual activities.
4. Find and eliminate obsolete rituals that do not serve your needs.
5. Approach your analysis with enthusiasm. Your attitude affects the results.
6. Make real changes. Avoid being superficial.

C. *Food Journal*

1. Review your Journal for *trends*:
   a. relaxed eating;
   b. thirty-minute time allotment;
   c. spacing between meals;
   d. proper nutrition to avoid hunger;
   e. proper nutrition to avoid "diet tricks."
2. Write before you eat.
3. Strive for accuracy. Strive for more success.

D. *Weight Chart*

1. Weigh yourself.
2. Mark your weight on the chart.
3. Make a connecting line to last week's weight mark.

E. *Time for Session 3*

One week, seven days, as usual.

SESSION 4

Easy Does It

For the past three weeks you have been challenging your old entrenched eating behavior patterns. Introducing change, in an effort to disrupt old patterns, is resisted by strong instinctive tendencies to keep things status quo. However, you are now ready to use your new constructive eating patterns to completely extinguish those old patterns.

This week's session will emphasize the finer points of change. You need no longer fear reverting to old behavior. In order to return to old eating habits now, you would have to buck the natural current, as opposed to being pulled back. That means simply that you would really have to work at eating improperly. Of course, you would not permit yourself to fall into that trap now.

Previous sessions on altering behavior patterns gave you some insight into the role of your environment in controlling your behavior. You discovered many areas that you will permanently rearrange.

At this time, you may be downright bored with food and with eating. If food is no longer your prime concern and eating has become a "bore," you are making anticipated progress. Stay bored with food until the tide turns, in a manner of speaking. Delay beginning each meal for one minute after sitting down, to further minimize any sense of emergency about eating. This is an additional required rule of eating behavior.

The Mannix Method is designed to train you to appreciate good food and to enjoy eating. Food is one of the marvelous treasures of the world. Pace yourself now, and don't let your temporary non-interest in food lead to skipping meals or to finding other activities to occupy your time while you are eating. You are undoubtedly feeling lighter and you are wearing some of the clothes that were stored in the back of your closet. Take pride in your accomplishment and work on this session with renewed enthusiasm. You are beginning to build on good patterns of behavior. Renew your commitment! Realize that it has been easier than you had anticipated and it will become easier and easier each and every day. You will finally possess all the finely sharpened tools for enjoying food, good health, and vitality.

MIRROR, MIRROR, ON THE WALL

Along with the new techniques that you learn, it is extremely important to reward yourself, so that you clearly register your progress. Begin to think thin. See yourself in the mirror as thinner and thinner. Visualize the beautiful *you* emerging from that packaging of fat. I suggest to all of my clients that they look at themselves disrobed in the mirror every day. Look through that fat and imagine what you really look like and how attractive you really are. Before long, the mirror will reflect what you are waiting to see. So begin looking now, and watch your better body emerge. As you look in the mirror every day—or better yet, as you look in the mirror twice each day—repeat to yourself, "I like myself without reservation and I am capable of doing anything that I choose to do." *I like myself without reservation.* That means that there is no more blame, no more guilt for being fat. You are now doing something about yourself, for yourself. You know that you are capable of doing anything you choose to do. You feel it. You see it! You are changing the circumstances that helped to make you fat. Once and for all time, you are meeting

the problem at the root level. Feel proud about your good judgment. You are your own best friend!

YOU HAVE A DREAM

Everyone who wants to be thin really wants something else.
Digest that! Everyone who wants to be thin really wants to be
thin so that he or she can do something else! What is it you really
want that being thin will make possible? When you analyze your
motivation and you understand it, you can work on that real
goal. You now know how to stay thin. You must stop being obsessed about losing weight. Devote more of your energy to
achieving your real rewards.

Make another list of some of the things that you consider the
rewards of being thin. Compare this list with your first one. What
do you look forward to now? Review the list and arrange those
rewards according to their importance to you. Choose one or
choose two of those rewards and write them on your weight
chart, or tape your top priorities across your mirror, or on the refrigerator door. Put them in the places that will keep those top
priorities in full view at a glance.

When tension or frustration triggers you to eat, flash your
thoughts to your real purpose. Ask yourself if eating will jeopar-
dize your dream! Think before you eat!

Maybe you really want to be thin to find a mate, or to improve
your sex life, or to wear beautiful attractive clothes, or to play
tennis or to go hiking. Perhaps you really want to lose weight to
be more like the people you admire, or to stop sweating, or
maybe just to really enjoy a day at the beach.

Make your list. Put time and thought into facing the real reasons for losing weight. Make those reasons your top priorities
now.

Today, I asked one of my clients why she thought she really
wanted to lose weight. In a mere ten seconds, she said, "I just
want to throw on a turtleneck top and a pair of jeans and not
have to go to the mirror to see if I look like a sausage in them—
which I always have. All of my clothes are designed to be attractive on their own merit. They do nothing to make me look attrac-

tive! I'm fed up with all of the hours that I spend camouflaging fat."

Another client says:

"I want to go out and dance and have some fun. I dance in my apartment alone now, and even with no one there to see me, I get depressed and I stop."

Another client reports:

"I have studied voice and opera for ten years. I'm ready to make singing my profession. But I am rejected for almost every part I audition for, because of my appearance. I want to lose weight so that I can pursue my career."

Still another client says:

"I know that I've been passed up for promotion in my company because I am fat. I do my job very well. My future depends on my losing weight—my whole future depends on my becoming presentable."

A salesman reports:

"It seems that all I do is sweat. Whenever I call on a customer, by the time I arrange my necktie, put on my jacket, and get up to the reception desk, I have sweated right through my shirt, and through the back of my jacket.

"My hand is wet when I shake hands and I continuously mop my brow during all of my interviews. I know that I could sell more if I could concentrate on selling. I can't stand it any longer."

Very often a definite decision to lose weight comes as the result of one particular incident. What was the incident that made you decide, once and for all, to do something about your weight? That incident usually holds within it the reason that really motivates you to become thin.

Discover your real purpose now that you are feeling better, and build your reward system with that as your goal. If you want to wear tight jeans and a sweater and not have to think about whether you look like a sausage, go out right now and buy those jeans and that great sweater. Hang them right in the front of your closet. Try them on every week to feel them getting closer and closer to your size. When you feel discouraged or tense, go to your closet and try your new outfit on. Let it remind you that you want to work hard at practicing your new eating habits.

If you want to be thin to play tennis or golf, and to be a part of that life-style, buy the equipment and the clothing that goes along with it. Begin to practice at home until the day when you are ready to go out to get really involved in the sport of your choice.

Everyone needs a dream! Everyone needs goals and rewards en route to a destination, whether it be to lose weight, to build a career, or to perfect a skill. We need to be rewarded at points along the way, or we may lose sight of our objectives. You know your goal. It is not to weigh a particular number of pounds, which is just a number signifying nothing. It is to achieve your greater goal! Find your deep reason for losing weight. You will find the rigors of reaching that goal easier when you understand your real deep-down purpose.

Food may be just a substitute for true emotional satisfaction. Realize your true emotional satisfaction, and you will find that your desire for excess food will vanish.

MAKE CHOICES

You are now eating in a more logical order and food is no longer your master. It is time to substitute healthy foods for some of your old favorites. It is also time to experiment with alternative activities to replace some of your old, inappropriate eating practices.

Food management is an exercise in planning just like the management of finances, household chores, or any of the other planning problems in our lives. Although all management procedures are problems in the sense that they must be solved in a logical manner to be effective, they need not be problems in the sense of being annoying. If you organize simple procedures logically and stick with them, the results will be surprising.

For instance, a friend of mine dislikes the details of paperwork, especially paying the bills and banking chores. The thought of paying bills and of balancing a checking account each month becomes torturous. But the bills must be paid, and accounts must be kept in order, so she devised a method to make the job easier and pleasanter. She pays each bill on the day she receives it. She balances her checking account on the day she receives her statement from the bank. She faces the jobs that she likes the least immediately, before they become monsters in her mind. Paying one bill at a time is like one step at a time. It minimizes the size of the dose. Ten or fifteen minutes of an unpopular chore is more palatable than hours of it at one time.

In a sense, you are losing weight in similar fashion by exercising small efforts with each exposure to food and to eating. The immediate task is your only consideration. You are never faced with too many changes to take care of all at once. You are learning to eat with appreciation. You are not on a diet!

To make your behavior modification most effective, your next step is to modify your attitude about food, especially food that has caused you the most difficulty.

For almost every damaging food, there is a healthy alternative that you can learn to prefer. It is part of modifying your behavior to permit yourself to change your attitudes about food. So look for foods that are healthy as a new way of life. Don't continue to dig your grave with your fork!

Choose the foods that you can enjoy. You won't change all of your problem foods, so don't punish yourself. Eat foods that you can't live without at appropriate times in your energy-demand style of eating. Try pizza, spaghetti, or baked potatoes for breakfast and feel sorry for everyone who diets. Enjoy the difference in tension.

Make some alternative choices in your activities around the house. Of all the causes for inappropriate eating at home, boredom heads the list. It is inexcusable to eat because you are bored when you can create other interesting activities to occupy your time and your thoughts.

You can change frustration and boredom to satisfaction and interest. Eating, as a release from boredom and from frustration, is a lazy choice. Digesting food is hardly a substitute for real emotional satisfaction. If you will channel some of your energy into finding some of your real needs, your search for unnecessary food will disappear. You must begin to examine your environment for activities other than the eating activity to capture your attention, so that you may avoid your old behavior of looking for food as a primary choice for satisfaction.

Don't look for magic activities that will automatically replace

the preoccupation you had with food. Rubbing magic lanterns is
not part of the Mannix Method. Instead, develop alternative activities that will keep you busy for as long as it takes to replace
your old habit of eating indiscriminately. Find something that
can command your attention for fifteen or twenty minutes. That
should be enough time for you to handle that irrational desire for
food. Break the chain of events that has always led to eating as a
substitute for some real emotional satisfaction.

Remember, food is not the problem. Eating is the problem. You
will find that any moderately interesting activity can be used to
replace the unrewarding one of eating. Please keep in mind that
although eating has been a substitute for real emotional satisfaction in your life, it has been very unsatisfying each time you used
it as a substitute. It produces immediate guilt and eventual dis-
comfort and embarrassment. Finding a really satisfying alternative activity may be surprisingly simple. It may be at your very
fingertips. Look around you!

The Mannix Method is designed to keep you shapely for the
rest of your life. There is no magic to this method. When you
have reached your weight goal using these simple techniques,
you may take all the credit, and rightly so. Do not lose sight of
the importance of keeping a positive attitude and actively pursu-
ing each new skill with renewed commitment and with enthusiasm.

List and review all of your interests. In addition to the activities that you are already familiar with, plan to explore some new
ones. Remember, no one technique in the Mannix Method is
earthshaking by itself. Everything works in harmony to build a
structure for a more satisfying life-style.

Most people associate sacrifice with diets. You are probably
waiting for the supreme effort to be required in the Mannix
Method. Believe it or not, there is no great sacrifice! This is the
show, so to speak, so put all you have into it now. Find some alternative activities that will hold your interest for a while so you
won't turn to food and to fat as the substitutes for real emotional
satisfaction.

"I tried a number of activities around my house as alternatives
to eating, but they all just reminded me that I was trying them to
forget about food," reported Marjorie Simms. "I finally realized

that these activities—reading, polishing silver, cleaning the fish tank—were all things I had always done just before or after eating. So I went out and I bought an inexpensive watercolor kit and some drawing paper to try my hand at painting. I had never tried painting before, but I knew that I had to find something totally different. For a six-dollar investment in supplies, my entire life has changed. I love to paint and I'm really good at it. I feel artistic all the time, and that applies to food too. I've hung my paintings in my dining room so I can enjoy them while I am enjoying my meals. I've never been so happy, nor so thin!"

"I've never been much for hobbies, but I was determined to find an alternative activity," client Albert Piper said. "We had this old grandfather clock that my wife's grandfather actually made and left to us. It never worked, so I thought that I would open it up and see if I could fix it. I had never tried anything like that before, and I wasn't too sure it would hold my interest. I was also a little afraid that it would frustrate me if I couldn't figure it out. I don't need more frustration after a long day at my job! I took the clock out to the garage after dinner one night and began taking it apart. That first night, I worked on it until my wife came out to remind me that it was after one o'clock in the morning. The time flew by and I hadn't thought of eating once. Every night for the next two weeks, I rushed out to the garage after work, skipping supper many times, to work on that clock."

"I wasn't bored as much as just angry that I had nothing to show for my life but a clean house, a fourteen-year-old son who didn't need me anymore, and a husband who thought of nothing but work. I was too fat to go out anywhere. After starting the Mannix Method, I realized that all of my friends were also fat and they enjoyed miserable company," Jane Hamilton said.

"I used to play tennis when I was younger and thinner, but that is out of the question now. That makes me angry. I hate to knit, and reading has always been coupled with a tray of snacks. I don't want to find an activity in the house. I am embarrassed to go out, and frankly, I don't have the strength very often to move. It made me angry just trying to find an alternative activity. I sat down and made a list of the things that had interested me in the past, and next to them I wrote a reason I was no longer interested in them. I found that I was so involved in writing the list and the reasons, the whole afternoon had gone by and my husband had come home from work. My son followed soon after. I had spent four hours writing the list, and I had even forgotten to prepare dinner. We went out to dinner that night. I was so preoccupied with the thought of having spent four hours at the kitchen table writing the list, never thinking of food, that I lost interest in dinner too.

"The next day, after everyone had left and the house was in order, I sat down again at the kitchen table, and I began writing about why I was fat and very angry. I wrote until I felt a little hungry. It was then lunchtime, and I had written for four hours again without a break. I put my writing aside and prepared a nice lunch, logged it in my Food Journal, and ate lunch at the dining-room table instead of the kitchen table, which now seemed to be reserved for my writing. After lunch I returned to writing and was occupied until suppertime. I wrote again after supper, and I wrote until I forced myself to stop so that I could relax in a nice hot bath to get tired for bed.

"I found a real emotional satisfaction in writing. Since then I have completed the Mannix program and have lost weight without difficulty. I will never get fat again because food doesn't interest me in the way that it used to. I am always practicing my new behavior techniques. Most important of all, I am busy writing. I've had some of my stories published in our local newspaper, and some are being considered by a couple of really prestigious magazines."

Food can be a substitute for real emotional satisfaction. Find that real satisfaction and your obsessive need for food will vanish. You handle food easily now, so pause to search for something to replace eating as a source of satisfaction.

"I thought I'd try something as obviously time-consuming as a jigsaw puzzle," says Martha Frieling. "I just poured out the contents of a jigsaw puzzle on a spare table and began fitting the pieces together. Every time I thought of snacking, I promised myself that I would first work on the puzzle for at least fifteen minutes. It really worked. My problem time was in the evening after supper. I would nibble all night and then sometimes I would even get up after I went to bed to nibble some more through the night. Every time that I went for the kitchen, I redirected myself to the puzzle. I soon found that I would spend more than just fifteen minutes with the puzzle, and I actually enjoyed the accomplishment of figuring out how the pieces fit. After working each time with the puzzle, I wasn't in the mood for eating anymore. I didn't know why, I didn't fight it—I just didn't eat.

"I knew that working on a jigsaw puzzle wasn't the answer to real emotional satisfaction for me, so I tried other activities every other time, hoping to hit upon one that would really capture my interest and allow me to grow. I came across an article in a magazine about macrame. I thought I'd give it a try and I went down to the local art-supply store to buy hemp and an instruction booklet. I didn't wait to have an urge to nibble. I began to weave knots right after dinner. Let me tell you, I found my real satisfaction. I have produced the most beautiful pieces of woven art that I have ever seen. I give macrame pieces to my family and friends for Christmas presents. I make them all with love and satisfaction. Every piece I finish weighs the pounds that my body would have been wearing if I hadn't made it. I can't tell you how important my hobby is to me."

"I've always wanted to play the trumpet," reports a physician client, "so I used this opportunity to develop an alternative activity. I rented a trumpet and began learning to play it. My family forced me to practice in the basement, but that didn't bother me. Every time that I felt an urge to snack, I would go down to the basement and practice for half an hour. I would then return to my usual evening work without the urge to eat. After a few months, I was actually getting good at playing the trumpet. I now plan on two half-hour practice sessions during my evenings of work at my desk. And I look forward to them just the way I used to look forward to cake and milk in the past."

Your alternative activities don't have to be continuing interests like the ones just mentioned. They may be things that must be done, like painting furniture or fixing the car. They may be cleaning projects that don't seem to ever get finished. They should be time-consuming projects that can replace your eating out of a sense of boredom and of frustration.

Make your list. Try the most available tasks first, or if you feel really motivated, go out and buy the supplies to begin a new project. You have thought of many things that you would like to try someday! The time is *NOW!*

DEEP RELAXATION

Boredom, frustration, pressure, disappointment, depression, and excitement are all familiar excuses for treating yourself to something to eat. You have now mastered some skills for controlling your eating during periods of tension. Now, you must work on controlling the *tension* itself.

Sit in a comfortable chair, close your eyes. Breathe deeply and slowly three or four times. Try to fill your abdomen with air. With each breath, exhale for fifteen seconds while you inventory and release the physical tension areas. Momentarily tense and then release your scalp. Do that by trying to lift, then drop, your ears. Move on to your forehead and then to your eyebrows. Tighten them for a second, then—*relax.* Next, tighten and then release your eyes, your face, and your jaw muscles. Move on to your neck and to your throat. Then go to your shoulders. Pull them up high behind your neck until they burn. Then let them drop. Let your arms hang heavy. Let gravity, the heavy pull from the earth's center, pull your arms down. They are too heavy to lift. Release your stomach muscles; work on every muscle in your stomach area. Then tighten your buttocks. Hold those muscles tight, tight, t-h-e-n release those tight muscles in your buttocks. Tighten those thigh muscles—hold them tight, hold them, hold them, t-h-e-n release the muscles in your thighs. Tighten the muscles in your calves. Tighten the calf muscles in the left leg, then in the right leg—all the muscles in the calves of both of your legs are tight, tight—then—release the muscles in both of your calves. Move on to your ankles, and then to your insteps. Tighten and then relax every muscle in your body all at once, tighten everything together as you take your second d-e-e-e-e-p breath. With your third and fourth breaths, try releasing all those areas without tightening them first. Pay close attention to your jaw muscles. Wiggle your lower jaw from side to side to release any possible tension there. The head and the neck areas are considered "where you live," in a manner of speaking.

Physical relaxation requires daily practice and patience. It is important to practice controlling tension. It is important to avoid old responses to tension and to frustration. You must break the old chains of behavior that result in eating when you are not hungry.

Allocate time every day of your life for deep relaxation. Some people include it in their starting routines, others make time in the day, and many prefer to wind down when day is done. It enhances living.

CRISIS CONTROL

Following are two quick crisis techniques that will help you to handle tension on the spot:

1. *Deep Breathing* Take the deepest breath you can hold. Hold it for a count of four. E-x-h-a-l-e very s-l-o-w-l-y, as though you were blowing up a balloon.

To practice a full breath, lie flat on your back on the floor, bed, or couch. Place your fingers just beneath your lowest ribs, then pant like a dog. That movement against your fingertips is made by the diaphragm function. To inflate your lungs to full capacity it is necessary to move the diaphragm out of the way so that the lungs can fill up at the bottom. The only direction for your diaphragm to move out of the way is down and out—toward your fingers. Practice a full deep breath lying down. Feel the diaphragm pushing against your fingertips. Then stand up and practice another full breath to experience the same pressure against your fingers. Be careful not to pull the diaphragm up into the rib cage by lifting your shoulders instead of pushing down and out.

If you don't feel pressure against your fingertips when you take a full breath while standing, go back to a horizontal position and practice it again. While you are lying down or bending over, the diaphragm is forced to move in the correct direction to fill your lungs to their capacity. Practice taking full deep breaths when lying down or bending over until you are able to duplicate the same movement of the diaphragm when you are standing up.

Whenever you feel yourself getting tense or having that old familiar urge to eat—STOP! Take a full deep breath. Hold it, hold it for four seconds. Now, s-l-o-w-l-y, using your back pressure, let your breath out for fifteen or twenty seconds. If the tension is great, fill your lungs two or three times. With each exhalation concentrate on releasing the tension in your neck and in your shoulders. Drop your shoulders. Feel your arms getting long and heavy as you exhale. Tell yourself to *relax*. Close your eyes. Concentrate on your neck and shoulders while releasing their tension.

After breathing deeply, concentrate on some unimportant object for a short spell, so that you can fix your new relaxed state before frustration builds again. It's just a matter of breaking a tension chain and redirecting your energy away from tightening your muscles again.

2. *Press the Tongue to the Roof of the Mouth* This is a relaxation technique that is useful for intensely anxious moments that need immediate control. Usually tension attacks the head and shoulder areas first. Clenched teeth and rigid tongue and lips are very obvious signs of the body in a state of tension, both physical and emotional.

When you experience severe tension, your head and your shoulders strain. You can relieve a good part of this tension by increasing the strain and then by releasing it deliberately. A very effective and simple way to do this is to press your tongue as hard as you can against the roof of your mouth for a count of ten. Then release the pressure slowly, releasing the strain around the ears, the eyes, the forehead, and then the neck and the shoulders. After practicing this exercise a few times, you will feel a natural progression of release in those areas. Try the suggested progression first, then vary it to meet your individual needs. At the end of this releasing procedure, make little air pockets in your cheeks, wiggle your jaw, and loosen the muscles in your whole face.

Both of these quick relaxation exercises will rescue your life when outside pressures are strangling you. You have usually turned to food to relieve pressure until now. Reassign your releasing procedures from eating to relaxing. Then manage the crisis causing your tension.

Volumes have been written about coping and about facing tension. With the success you are enjoying with the Mannix Method and the attendant weight loss, your self-confidence has been growing. You are strong and in control of everything in your life. You are no longer the victim of your environment. You are able to cope with many of the pressures around you. You may even find that familiar pressures and daily tensions are diminishing with your body measurements.

These two relaxation techniques will help you to deal with tension instantly without immediately turning to food. Try one or both of these techniques when you want to relax. Use deep breathing often through the day. Take a deep breath before every activity. It will refresh you. You will start each new task with your undivided attention. Use the "tongue" technique for the more acute moments of tension. After pressing and slowly releasing your tongue, take a deep breath and get the most from combining techniques.

Pressing the tongue tends to relax the nerves and face muscles, while deep breathing produces a physical relaxation by lowering the heart rate and the blood pressure. Use both techniques frequently throughout the day and always in emergencies. They will help to allow you to cope without food.

FOOD JOURNAL

Review your Food Journal for the week. Your total eating time should be very consistent at this point. You show thirty minutes for every meal except when you have been unable to finish all of your food and have left part of the meal on the plate.

Starting now, with this session, *leave two bites* on your plate every time that you eat. If you have been eating everything, each bite at every meal, and of course clocking the full thirty minutes, prepare two extra bites at each meal so that you may continue to eat as much as you have been, but will now have two extra bites to leave.

The purpose of this procedure is to allow you to learn that you don't have to consume every bit of food on your plate. Your appestat must decide when you are satisfied and you are finished eating, not the size of the portion that you are served. Your appestat control has been sorely neglected until now and is even now only dimly sensed. Reinforce its functioning by visually experiencing that all of your food has not been devoured, and lo and behold, you feel full and satisfied!

Also check your Food Journal for any unnecessary snacks or idle nibbling. Remember, *if you eat, make it worth your while.* No snacks: Eat only meals.

SUMMARY

This week has been important in your progress. You have finally erased old eating behavior and replaced it with new patterns. This week is the first week for leaning completely on your new learning.

Be not harsh or timid, but like Goldilocks and the porridge, be "just right." Don't challenge your strengths and your weaknesses. Just depend on your new behavior with confidence.

Help yourself by choosing good foods and interesting spare-time activities. Put your every effort into another week of training.

Your big efforts for this session are to overcome your disenchantment with food and to transfer your energy to constructive, interesting activities. Find activities as alternatives for eating. Practice relaxation techniques that will help you to cope with daily tension and frustration, and that will enhance living.

Be in control! Expect that you will be in control! Know that you will be in control! Have faith in yourself, in your ability to make plans and to follow them. You are on your way! Welcome to the sunny side of life!

Commit yourself by signing the following contract.

Remember that this is a point of honor—a private obligation to yourself:

CONTRACT

With my initials below, I pledge my best effort in following each and every step in the Mannix Method described in Session _____4_____ for the next 7 days.

Initial: _____

Date: _____

HIGHLIGHTS

A. Think Thin.

1. Disrobe every day in front of the mirror. Watch your new self emerge.
2. Say to yourself, *loud and clear,* "I like myself without reservation. I am capable of doing anything that I choose to do!" Say that every day in front of your mirror.
3. Delay beginning to eat for one minute.

B. Everyone Who Wants to Be Thin Really Wants Something Else.

Everyone who wants to be thin really wants something else that being thin will bring about!

1. Make a list of the rewards of being thin. List the things that you are looking forward to.

2. Decide on the goals that your being thin will help you to realize. Write them in bold letters across your mirror, on your weight graph, and on the refrigerator door.

C. Understand Your Real Emotional Satisfactions.

Work for real emotional satisfaction instead of the false satisfaction that overeating provides.

D. Plan Ahead.

1. Learn that food management is a budgeting problem.
2. Plan ahead. Organize your approach to food.
3. Modify your attitudes about food. Replace high-calorie-food stuffers with healthy, nourishing foods.
4. Prefer healthy food. Love life.
5. Remove empty foods that you can do without. Have the ones that you can't live without for breakfast.

E. Find Alternative Activities.

1. Don't eat because you are bored or frustrated.
2. Find "other" activities to hold your attention.
3. List activities that you already enjoy, that are readily available.
4. List new activities that you may want to try. Get the necessary supplies.
5. Remember, food is not the problem: Eating is.
6. Commit yourself to your alternate activity with enthusiasm. Make it work for you!

F. Learn Relaxation Techniques.

1. Deep relaxation: Practice daily.
2. Deep breathing will relax you physically and help you to get control. Then face the music.
3. Tongue pressure against the roof of your mouth releases tension in the face and shoulders. Rely on this for immediate relief from acute tension.

G. Food Journal

1. Review your records.
2. Check total eating time.
3. Always leave two bites—on every course, every plate, every time. Don't run out of food.

H. Weight Chart

1. Weigh yourself. Record your weight.
2. Expect a weight loss of 2 pounds.

I. Time

One week is assigned to all sessions.

SESSION 5

Coming Out

Have you noticed that you are changing your life-style? Food is no longer your major consideration and serenity seems to prevail almost to the point of monotony.

This is the time for you to venture out of the cocoon that you have spun around yourself for your security. Look for dinner invitations and try some unfamiliar restaurants. Take some chances and anticipate possible pitfalls. Be ready to control situations and to survive!

It is no easy matter to be the victor in any battle. Losing weight permanently is not easy. You must be the victor in small skirmishes to survive the main battle.

Right now you may be feeling a little fatigued. You have completed one month of bucking old eating behaviors. You have observed your behavior more thoughtfully than ever before, and are watching an old familiar friend disappear right before your eyes. Perhaps you feel a kind of melancholy. Even though that old friend has caused you heartache and embarrassment, you have still learned to depend on your fat friend to give you comfort. It is natural to grieve when we lose something or become separated. Be aware of your loss and appreciate the dynamics of separation. You are permitting yourself to emerge from your cage. Appreciate your opportunity!

You are becoming thin. It doesn't really matter how long it will take you—you are in process, in the process of getting thin and of achieving that special goal that you have dreamed about. Do not fear leaving the security of your fat.

Uncertainty usually frightens us. But leaving a warm nest for unknown places can be an adventure when it is planned. However, no matter how we plan, we still feel anxious. Don't look back! You have set your goal! Keep your eyes looking forward, hold your head high, and stay on course!

You may pause for a moment to bid farewell to your prison cell. Reminisce today if you must, but move on.

Every now and then we read about a prisoner who is returned to society after being held captive for many years, only to commit an obvious crime and to be returned to prison. He is returned to the horrible condition of imprisonment that he had become dependent on. His spirit was too broken to accept a challenge, whatever the pleasures and the prizes. He was frightened of change with all the advantages that it might bring!

I remember also when the television star Jack Paar rescued a number of African lions by having them shipped to a zoo in the United States so that they could be properly cared for. When the crates with the lions were delivered to the zoo after a lengthy voyage with numerous delays, and the doors of the crates were opened to free the lions, none of the animals would move out of their confinement. They had grown "crate trained." They had undoubtedly been lured and then forced into those crates, but they had learned to find comfort within those four walls. They were secure in knowing their limits. Cry for those trapped beasts. Cry for the prisoner who copes better in captivity. Cry for yourself if you cannot face life without fat!

Recognize your goals and pocket your fears. Your rewards will be great. The unknown will become comfortably familiar in a wink. Change your dull routine by making breakfast dates with friends and with business associates.

Susanna Hernes, a thirty-five-year-old textile designer and a client of mine, explains how she changed routines:

"I'm one of the top executives in an international textile firm. During my working day, which has always seemed to take all of my waking hours, I meet with executives from other large corporations to discuss business deals involving millions of dollars. The textile industry is comprised mostly of men. Meetings are always out of town for one of us. It is part of my job either to be hostess to a visitor or to be a guest when I am out of town. That usually means rich lunches and many elaborate dinners.

"Well, now that I'm getting thin and attractive, I am very aware of my eating, as you may well imagine. So I have decided to try hosting at breakfast meetings. I flatly refuse dinner invitations. It has worked out marvelously. No one expects an invitation to breakfast, so they never refuse. Some of the most charming restaurants in town serve the most fabulous breakfasts. Breakfasts are delicious and seem to be much more appreciated than dinner meals. The time of the day is perfect. Our meetings are fresh and spontaneous. I'm so glad that I tried it. I'm known now for being the most attractive breakfast hostess in the business. Of course, that's a joke! But it is a mark of distinction and a bit of fun in transactions that can become very dull and flat."

Change your style of living! Break out of your crate and try new things. Invite a friend out to breakfast. There are many very special cozy restaurants in your town. With each breakfast date, you will be reinforcing your new eating behavior, and be reaping rewards at the same time.

Lunch is the next-best meal for experimenting with your new eating behavior. Instead of lunch simply being the meal that follows breakfast, make it a celebration as often as you can. Forget the mundane sandwich! Enjoy creating an interesting treat or try eating out at some delightful restaurant. If you are a working person with a definite lunchtime, try various restaurants close to your office. Lunch at some of the elegant restaurants in town may not be as costly as you expect. Most very expensive dinner restaurants serve surprisingly reasonable lunches. Live a little! If you are eating lunch out, try to afford a better place once or twice each week. It will make you feel luxurious and will allow you to experiment with different kinds of foods around people who take eating very seriously.

If you eat lunch at home, vary your choice of foods. The old standbys, tuna fish and chicken, can get pretty dull if you eat them every day. Cottage cheese can hold your attention only for a very short time. So get involved! Cook interesting foods for lunch. Invite friends for lunch and show off! Also think of preparing dinner meals for breakfast. Treat yourself to the best life has to offer. You are a most important person!

Going out to dinner at the homes of friends or at restaurants is fun and can be harmless. Just plan ahead. Be ready to control your environment instead of being controlled by your environment. Be the master, not the victim.

If you are invited out to a friend's house for dinner, call ahead and explain to your host or to your hostess that you are not eating protein or starch for supper at this time. Tell them that you don't want to appear unappreciative if you leave the entree—that is, if the entree is protein or starch. Any of your friends will appreciate your kindness and will usually prepare vegetables and sufficient salad to accommodate you.

If you call early enough your host or your hostess may be challenged to prepare an entree without protein or starch that everyone will enjoy. Or if you prefer to keep your plans private, just become an expert at moving the food around on your plate. Eat the things that you can and play with the rest.

At restaurants order a vegetable or a salad dish. Order your favorite cut of meat and tell the waiter before he serves it that you will be taking your meat home with you. Ask him to be kind enough to keep it in the kitchen until you are ready to leave. Most waiters will bend over backward to please. Don't tell the waiter what to do, ask for his help. The experienced waiter will understand. You will enjoy dinner, and can eat your protein for breakfast at home.

Feel free to order things in restaurants that are not on the menu. Restaurants expect special requests. Order just exactly what you want! If the waiter is smart, he will know that if he extends himself he will earn a larger tip, so be assured that he is on your side. Request what you want. You are paying for it, so assert yourself. Don't be timid about what you buy for your money.

The point is to venture out into our great big wonderful world! Vary your eating conditions. Welcome new eating situations. Control what you eat, at any place that you eat it. Be kind to yourself! If a waiter puts bread on the table, ask him to remove it. You did not ask for it! If potatoes are served on your plate, ask the waiter to remove the potatoes. You did not ask for them. If your neighbor drops by with a piece of pie that she has just baked, thank her for being thoughtful but ask her to take the pie back. Tell her that you will look forward to it sometime in the future—in your thin future.

You are not a victim of your environment. You must control your environment. Make it serve you! Choose what you will eat or what you will not eat. Don't discipline yourself with food. LIVE A LITTLE!

LIQUIDS

One of the first questions clients ask is whether they will be asked to drink certain quantities of water with the Mannix Method.

It is unnatural to force ingestion, whether it be food or water. Your body regulates fluids, so try to understand your body needs. Learn some of the facts.

The body produces four and a half pounds of water for every four pounds of dissolved fat. If you don't keep the water moving, theoretically you can gain weight while you are losing fat. Of course that doesn't actually happen, but remember that you must keep the water flowing through and out of your system.

Where do the lost pounds go? They must be excreted through the bowels and the urinary tract. Fluids facilitate excretion. Fluids facilitate weight loss!

Water is the very best fluid. It leaves behind the least amount of residue to be processed and to be eliminated with the fat. In a sense, other fluids compete with the fat to be eliminated. Learn to appreciate water. It is your good friend.

Stop drinking soft drinks all through the day. Sugared soft drinks are unnecessary consumption of calories that should be obtained from healthy food. Sugar-free soft drinks are low in calories, but they should be taken with caution. The continuous sipping of soft drinks keeps you tasting all day long. Reserve tasting for meals. Don't be involved with food all through your day. Fruit juices and milk should be considered food.

Remember, too, that caffeine is a drug. It is addictive! Coffee, cola, cocoa, and regular tea will give you a momentary lift and may even avert rising hunger for a short time, but the letdown will leave you hungrier, more confused, depressed, more anxious, and will undermine the control that you have been working so hard to develop. If you are a heavy consumer of any of these beverages you may want to eliminate them slowly from your diet. Expect some feelings of withdrawal, however. Fatigue is the most common withdrawal symptom. Other symptoms are apathy, feelings of hopelessness, and mild depression. Plan carefully before you completely eliminate any of these drugs.

This is probably as good a time as any to discuss alcohol. Many drinkers are hoping not to have to give up alcohol in order to lose weight and to gain control of their eating behavior. If you are keeping up with the program and you are losing weight and are still drinking alcohol, more power to you! If your weight loss is slow, however, or even nonexistent, and you are still drinking alcohol, you must reevaluate the role that drinking plays in your life.

Alcohol provides empty calories. There is no food value to the calories in alcohol. Alcohol isn't even digested the way food is digested. It is addictive, like sugar, and it goes directly into the bloodstream.

Estimate roughly a hundred empty calories for every portion of whiskey, beer, or wine. The exact caloric comparison is irrelevant. (One hundred calories, more or less, are consumed with every ounce of alcohol, glass of wine or beer.) Mixed drinks are usually more than one ounce, and most wine glasses hold more than the usual four ounces. Beer bloats your organs in addition to being higher in calories.

One of my clients, an attractive young businessman with very little weight to lose, couldn't seem to budge a pound off after he had quickly lost five pounds at the beginning of the program. His Food Journal showed a gin and tonic or two at lunch and two or three more before his supper. After a few weeks it was apparent that he had to examine his drinking habits if he wanted to lose any more weight. His total calories in cocktails for each day were a staggering 1200. He was eating sensibly, to be sure, but 1200 cocktail calories a day absolutely defeated any progress that he could ever make.

A possible way to treat the added alcohol calories is to save those calories from your meals that day. For instance, if you know on a Saturday morning that you will be having a few drinks that evening, trim those calories off your meals. Eliminate the starch at breakfast, or have fish for lunch instead of steak, or pass up the fruit after lunch. A little economy at all of your meals may balance those drinks that night. A few drinks every now and then should be permissible if you wish!

WALKING

You are ready for some physical activity at this point in your journey. It is necessary to keep your body limber and your blood circulating in order for your body to function properly. Aside from maintaining the body beautiful, physical movement is indispensable for staying young.

Disciplined exercise is impractical for most of us because of the dedication that it requires. But walking a short distance each day is certainly possible. Walking is as valuable as many of the more strenuous forms of physical exertion. As a matter of fact, as far as burning calories is concerned, walking is closely equivalent to jogging.

Starting today, plan a short walk sometime during your day. Your walk need not be long nor rapid. Walk as far as you wish and walk no farther than is pleasant for you. Use the time to revel in the nice feeling that you have in moving with more ease than you used to. Enjoy the day, the trees, the birds. Think of nothing but yourself and your surroundings. Feel your legs move, swing your arms, study the movement of your head. Walk for only as long as you can concentrate on your walking.

Add a walk to your commitment. Start with one single block. That will not take too much of your time. But find the time to walk sometime during your day. It is not enough to walk up and down an office corridor twelve times a day. Go out for a walk every day with the same commitment that you exercised in logging your Food Journal before you ate.

This is another of those commitments that may seem to be an effort at first, but will develop into one of the wonderful pleasures of your day. It is all the exercise that you will ever need to do. Develop it slowly.

Allot the rest of this week to adjusting your new schedule. If you have to rush through your walk any day this week, consider yourself in transition, and view the week as a trial week for including your walk. Next week, you should have a definite time set aside for walking. Permit only the most severe weather conditions to interfere.

You will never have to feel guilty again about an exercise program. Walk at your own pace for your own distance to the beat of your own drummer! Enjoy your freedom!

IMAGING

Imaging is a daydreaming procedure that can be used to reduce the tension that causes overeating. Imagine yourself in a place where you feel totally safe and secure. This is a procedure that is used extensively with people who are the victims of phobias. There are people who suffer a fear of flying in planes, of riding elevators, or of being confined in closed rooms. There is fear of dogs, snakes, water, machinery noises, and even phobic fear of the out-of-doors, of open space. The fear of the dark has been very successfully controlled with this "mind tripping" exercise called imaging.

Now that you understand and practice deep relaxation, relax deeply and let your mind drift away to a scene that brings you comfort and peace. Is it a childhood vacation spot? A trip to some wooded place? Is it a sunny day at a familiar beach, perhaps with cliffs jutting up in the background to protect you from the wind? A snowed-in family weekend? Or do you want to create the perfect spot from several places and times? Be careful not to put any people into your scene. Just keep it for yourself. Other people in your scene may destroy some of the sense of peace. They may change that place as your sanctuary. Keep it for yourself alone, as you want it, in every minute detail. Slowly, s-l-o-w-l-y, let your mind drift away. Equip your sanctuary with every possible detail. Is the air cold? Is it hot? Or is it just exactly right? What are you wearing? What does the ground under your feet feel like? Use all of your senses. Are there any familiar odors? Are there any sounds that bring peace to your sanctuary? Is it daytime? Is it dusk? Is it dark?

Notice every little significant detail. Turn around in your sanctuary scene, so that you may examine the things that surround you—in back of you, in front of you, at both of your sides. Are you standing? Sitting? Walking? What are you doing? Do you feel the peace? Are you in love? How old are you? Feel every sinew in your body, your thin agile body! Feel how healthy you are. Feel how strong you are! Live—in your sanctuary. Go there! Experience your sanctuary!

After you have made yourself aware of everything in your scene, and have relaxed and experienced the tranquility and security of your sanctuary, s-l-o-w-l-y take another deep breath. As you exhale, open your eyes and be sensitive to tension points. Then get up s-l-o-w-l-y and e-a-s-i-l-y. You are now ready to return to your usual schedule. Carry the quietness of your daydream with you when you resume your daily chores. Retain the sensitive scrutiny that you used in your scene. Look around you, observe the things around you, be aware of the things around you—the air, sounds, odors. Be aware of yourself, thin under your clothes. Uncover your own real thin body as you think about it, right now. The "thin you" is in the process of thinning, of emerging, of becoming the you in your sanctuary.

Here is one person's account of daydreaming:

"I closed my eyes, relaxed all tension spots, and with my third breath reached the top of the clay cliff that overlooked the ocean. In the distance, the robin's-egg-blue sky met a deep, deep, green ocean. That meeting line was the edge of this marvelous world that was all mine.

"The sun glistened on the water in wide streaks. I walked down the road to the foot of the cliffs to go to my beach. I made a path through the brush on the sand dunes, through beach-plum bushes and reeds. As I walked, my sandaled feet were buried in the warm, shifting sands. In moments I was on the white clean beach sheltered by the pastel-colored clay cliffs. I removed my sandals and threw them to the side. I listened to the rhythm of the waves breaking on the beach as the saltwater spray perfumed the air. There were no sounds but the pounding of the breaking waves and the occasional *caw, caw* of a swooping, graceful gray-and-white sea gull.

"I turned my face up to the warm sun with my eyes closed so that I could thaw. The air moved ever so slightly around my head to mix with heat and spray and magic sunlight.

"I walked to the base of the cliffs, feeling the sand hotter and hotter beneath my feet. I found a perfect place to rest my back, and when I sat down, a little movement on my part made a perfectly contoured seat.

"I stretched my legs and relaxed my body. A feeling of peace crept through my being."

Imaging will change your mood and slow your pace. After you practice it a few times and learn to eliminate extraneous thoughts from your sanctuary, you will be ready to use the exercise to calm yourself, and to strengthen your purpose. If you become upset and think about eating to heal your wounds, try imaging. One moment's pleasure of mouth stuffing cannot match your sanctuary for sheltering you. Life brings many disappointments. Eating in response to disappointment just adds more disappointment. It's a false solution. Instead, conjure an imaging scene that makes you feel safe and peaceful and good. Use your sanctuary to ease yourself out of stress situations that may trigger inappropriate responses. Create your own peaceful environment even as things seem to be crumbling around you. You can revitalize yourself in this way anywhere, as you rub your magic lantern. The more expert you become at imaging, the more complete your concentration will become and the more quickly you will be able to clear your thoughts and command confidence. Concentration is the magic in imaging. Shift your concentration from the things that lead you to respond inappropriately to thoughts that give you enough time to gain control of the situation. You will then be able to redirect your efforts. Eating as a solution will seem quite ridiculous to you. You will be able to remove yourself from stress; you will handle stress. You will cope with the situation intelligently.

How many times have you passed your own street or missed your turnoff on the highway because you were preoccupied with other thoughts? Have you ever put the milk back in the cupboard and the salt shaker in the refrigerator? One person had a habit of putting the mail into the freezer. The power of concentration is extraordinary. Use it in a positive way to soothe and to caress, not in a negative way to worry, to regret, and then to feel guilt.

FOOD JOURNAL

Review your Food Journal. Last week you were instructed to leave two bites of your food on the plate each time you ate. Review last week's entries to see if you were able to do that at each meal.

This week, in the column labeled Food/Amount in your Food Journal, record the amount of food that you left on your plate in addition to the amount of food that was served. For example, if you leave just two bites, record that. If you leave one fourth or perhaps one half of some of your meals, record that amount in the column designated for amount. This kind of record will give you a rather accurate idea of the amount of food that you actually consumed.

You will use your Food Journal for four more weeks. Try very hard not to become lazy about keeping these records. Record your information clearly and correctly. If you should happen to forget to bring your Journal home from the office, or vice versa, write your information on a piece of paper until you can transfer it to your Journal. Keep it as carefully as you keep your checkbook. Guard against permitting protein back into your supper meals. There will be changes in a few weeks, but until then stay with an evening meal that has no protein and no starch.

The Food Journal is a valuable tool for you. It may be getting a little repetitious at this point, but you must maintain your resolve to keep your records carefully. Know that practice makes perfect! It is to your advantage to keep the Food Journal religiously until it is discontinued. Don't become careless.

SUMMARY

Now that the excitement of making new commitments is wearing off, guard against undermining your success with self-pity and with the anxiety attendant on losing an old friend. You were familiar with your old, familiar, cumbersome, fat self. You are on your own on new and exciting terrain. Embrace the past with a passing glance and look to the future with courage.

You are no longer trapped in those old familiar surroundings. Remember your depression? Remember the disappointment that you lived with every day? Remember when you pulled your shirt down over your fat body to hide it? Remember when you used your clothing for privacy? Remember when you could actually hold a handful of your extra body tissue? Remember your disgust? Your despair? Your anger? Your envy? Now, realize your dream!

Get out of all your hiding places! Get out of your house! Live like a normal person—like most other people. Learn to be comfortable. Practice liking yourself! Find new restaurants, explore new stores, make new friends. Shed your old self and become free!

Commit yourself by signing the following contract.

Remember that this is a point of honor—a private obligation to yourself:

CONTRACT

With my initials below, I pledge my best effort in following each and every step in the Mannix Method described in Session ____5____ for the next 7 days.

Initial: _____

Date: _____

Highlights

A. Coming Out

1. It is normal to feel a little discouraged when discarding familiar things, be they good or bad.
2. It is normal to feel some fear about the unknown, the unfamiliar.
3. It is good to look ahead. Enjoy the challenge.
4. You must get out of your crate. Find new ways. They are better.
5. You must plan ahead. Control your environment.
6. You must assert yourself. Ask for the food that you want.
7. Try to make your meals interesting and fun. Pleasure is a freedom song!

B. Fluids

1. Don't force water. Your body regulates its need for fluid.
2. However, water is the purest and most easily handled fluid.
3. Fluids must flow through the body to eliminate fat.
4. Eliminate drinking soft drinks all through the day. Avoid continuous consumption.
5. Never drink sugared soft drinks.
6. Caffeine is addictive. It changes your blood-sugar levels.
7. Alcohol is metabolized like sugar. It has empty calories. It changes blood-sugar levels.

C. Walking

1. Walk every day.
2. Experiment with the time of day for your walk and with a comfortable distance.
3. Be aware of your body movement. Enjoy the freedom. Enjoy the environment! Enjoy your world.

D. Imaging

1. Reduce tension with daydreaming skills.

   2. Picture a sanctuary for shelter and security.
   3. Use relaxation skills to drift to your scene.
   4. Use all of your senses in your scene. Remember the details.
   5. Alter your mood and your pace with *imaging.*
   6. CONCENTRATE.

E. Food Journal

   1. Review.
   2. Begin to record the amount of food left on your plate.
   3. Maintain consistency.
   4. Continue to avoid protein and starch for supper.

F. Weight Chart

   1. Weigh yourself and graph a mark corresponding to your weight on the chart.
   2. Your graph will show a steady declining trend.

G. Time For Session 5

Use one full week for Session 5, as with all sessions.

SESSION 6

SECOND WIND

The work in Session 6 represents a continuation of the basic skills and techniques learned and practiced through the first five sessions. The changes and the additions in this session are rather subtle and perhaps less dramatic in terms of demonstrating immediate differences. You will be moving from the mechanics of behavior modification to an emphasis on psychological support. Continue to practice your learned skills with diligence. This session will provide additional reinforcement.

Long-distance runners tell of running an appointed distance anticipating a "second wind" to become revitalized. The second wind prepares them for running the rest of the distance. This second wind represents the time when the body is supplied with additional oxygen to meet the needs of continuing stress. Until that second wind, the body is being strained. Oxygen cannot be provided fast enough. Breathing becomes heavier and faster and the heart pumps faster. The heat produced from all of this activity becomes more intense. As the body strains from running, the supply system is just a little behind the demand. It is then that runners begin to experience fatigue. At this fatigue point they

119

begin to look for that second wind. The second wind represents the supply meeting the demand. When the demand for oxygen is met, runners report that they can then continue on almost indefinitely. At that point of fatigue, they also all report feelings of weakness and thoughts of losing the race. They keep running during that low point because they are familiar with those feelings and they anticipate their second wind. There is that moment, however, when each runner reviews his physical self to reassure himself that he can keep running.

You are now approaching your "second wind." You are probably feeling fatigued. You feel strain because you are moving toward your "second wind." You must now have faith in your ability to reach higher, to breathe that one breath that will be the beginning of your "second wind." This reach will take you the whole distance, despite any obstacles. Supply will match demand! Be patient. Believe in yourself! You have come a long way with great success. You may expect more and more of yourself. Your "second wind" will take you the whole distance.

CHEATING

The dictionary defines cheating as "the act of deceiving." Cheating suggests using trickery that escapes observation. It involves the deliberate perversion of the truth to fool "someone else."

It is in fact a concept that has no value in the Mannix Method of controlling behavior. The word may therefore be eliminated from your vocabulary and from your thoughts. Let us analyze why it has no meaning for you.

The Mannix Method is based on a *know thyself* philosophy. In order for you to alter your behavior and to build new patterns of behavior, you have been trained in the art of careful observation and the analysis of your own behavior. You were directed to recognize inner and environmental cues to eating. You have been trained to understand real goals. There is no one to deceive, no authority figure to fool, no "other" person to punish.

The Mannix Method is a method of control based on self-discovery and self-acceptance. It provides opportunity for you to be in touch with yourself so that you may reach for the dignified special person that you are. You are trained to face yourself, assert yourself, and enjoy freedom.

You have been trained to understand "normal" behavior. The word "normal" means that which is not unusual. It is not unusual to have an urge for a particular food every now and then. You are sufficiently skilled by this session to permit yourself some flexibility. Remember food is not the problem; *eating* is the problem. So with the full knowledge of what you do, why you are doing it, and when you may do it, enjoy that urge. You are *master* enough not to make it a *habit*.

It is about four inches from your lips to your swallow. Never forget that tasting is a very brief pleasure. The price, wearing those unnecessary calories on your body, may be foolishly expensive.

PLATEAUS

It is normal and not unusual to experience one or more periods of minimal or perhaps no weight loss with any attempt at losing excess body fat. The body needs time to adjust to a changing metabolism. The body also tends to retain water periodically after emptying fat cells.

Plateaus are discouraging if your only goal is to lose weight. Changing body proportion and body size would be a much more rewarding goal. While your weight stabilizes on plateau, you will still be diminishing size and feeling thinner.

If you have hit a plateau, be encouraged by the loose clothes. Appreciate your new image in the mirror every day. Avoid being negative. Anyone can despair and be discouraged. The "new you" can rise above external cues for triggering your behavior. You have chosen a new life-style. You are your own master. Choose to be a positive force in your own life.

DOWN WITH TRICKS

You need no longer invent "tricks" to fool yourself. Years of dieting have probably equipped you with dozens of inappropriate "tricks" to fool yourself into eating less. Let's examine some of those tricks and eliminate them. Let's substitute some dependable, sensible techniques instead.

First of all, don't weigh your food to determine how much you will eat. You have finished insulting yourself. You know what a small portion of food looks like. Because you have been using thirty minutes for each of your meals, you have developed the most dependable monitor of all. You have developed your appestat. You need not guess anymore. You feel how much food your body can comfortably handle. There is a record in your head about how much food you are able to consume comfortably. Rely on that information when you serve portions at your meals. Serve enough to meet your needs. Listen to your inner mechanism of hunger control. Respond responsibly. Respond intelligently.

The idea of using small plates and crowding them with food, to make believe, is child's play. It is rather a silly game. Too much food on a small plate may create a sense of emergency and may just influence you to want to eat faster. Crowding—crowding anything—tends to make us feel tense. An open, nicely arranged plate of food pleases the eye. Please all of your senses to really enjoy eating.

Continue to prepare all portions in the kitchen and bring plates to the table. Do not serve food at the table from serving dishes. If you want more food, return to the kitchen to get it. The inconvenience of leaving the table and going back to the kitchen may be enough disruption to make you pause to think it over. You may realize that you are not really hungry enough for more food.

Placing serving dishes on the table is an invitation to overeat. Opportunity creates temptation. Don't ever challenge your resolve unnecessarily.

Do you really want to test your appestat to learn portion control? Prepare a dinner salad large enough for four people. Sit down to the entire salad one evening at supper. Eat slowly, observing all behavior rules. Take intermissions whenever you feel that they are appropriate. Eat until you are satiated. You will have to rely on your appestat to say, "Stop! Stop!" The salad should be too large for you ever to be able to consume it in one sitting. There will be no question about portion control with this exercise. You are equipped with *stop* signals. Obey them!

DON'T LINGER BUT WAIT

Don't linger at the table after you have eaten. Move to another room to converse with friends and with family. Or get busy with one of your home projects. Clean the kitchen thirty minutes or more after you have left the table. Thirty minutes affords the time to quiet your eating mechanism. When you go back to doing the dishes, food will seem more repulsive than tempting.

A client, Florence Peterson, says:

"I was always afraid that I would continue nibbling after my supper meal. That had been my habit until now. The fear of eating after an adequate supper paradoxically drove me right straight back to eating. I just never seemed to be finished with my meal. I came up with a great solution that has worked for me every time. Right after my supper, I leave the table. I go directly to the living room to read a book. I make a point of reading for thirty minutes before doing anything else. When the time is up, I have completely lost the desire to eat. It's like a deprogramming time. I can then go back to the kitchen, put the food away, and clean up without being tempted to eat a bite!"

Eating is an intense activity. We try to minimize the intensity with the two intermissions during your meals. Any intense situation has momentum that carries over after the activity is finished. Anger, fear, and keen anticipation are intense feelings that remain with us after stimuli have been removed. There is a need to wind down and to put things back into their proper perspective.

If you have difficulty getting over the intensity of eating, move on to another engrossing activity immediately for at least thirty minutes. Reading is very helpful. It soothes and at the same time it demands your concentration. Choose something that absorbs your attention!

FOOD JOURNAL

Review your Food Journal for this week. Your Journal is on-

the-spot feedback of your success in controlling your eating behavior. Continue to write everything you eat *before* you eat it.

YOU'RE ONLY HUMAN

Your skills thus far in the Mannix Method have been designed
to eliminate indiscriminate eating and to develop appropriate
eating patterns. The combined use of all of your learned skills
will put you in control of your eating and of your weight. Understand the external cues that influence you to think about food.
You have really been learning to be sensitive to the negative
forces that enslave you! *Know thyself!* Eliminate the obvious.
Change your responses to false cues. Change the situations that
trigger undesirable chains of behavior.

Remember, don't quench all of your urges all of the time.
There are times when you may want to have some particular
food that pleases. It may not be an externally cued suggestion.
There will be occasions when your body will demand certain nutrients (food craving is not always psychological). Analyze all
your unusual food desires in light of your body needing additional vitamins or minerals. Exercise choice. Decide to eat or decide not to eat.

Margot Hannon reports: "It had been one of my favorite habits
to go to the movies every Sunday afternoon. I've been doing that
for more than two years, ever since I moved into the city from my
family's home upstate. I was doing very well with behavior modification and had lost most of the weight that I wanted to lose. I
was very proud of my control.

"All of a sudden this winter I was coming home from my Sunday matinee and I felt a strong desire to make some lemon meringue pie. The first time that that happened I didn't pay too
much attention. I had had urges for inappropriate things before
and I found that those urges usually passed quickly. But it happened again the following Sunday, and then again the next
week. It took longer and longer to get over the urge that I had for
lemon pie each week. I was frightened by this uncontrolled desire to eat something that I would normally choose not to eat.
The next time it happened, I was really upset. I suppose I blew
the whole thing out of proportion by doubting my ability to con-

trol the situation. I didn't want to eat any pie, but I felt that the urge was almost too strong to disregard. I tried to relax by doing some deep breathing. I closed my eyes and I began purposely to think about lemon meringue pie. I felt that this uncontrolled urge was tied up with the idea of the pie itself. It was my last try before I would give in and I knew it.

"I pictured the pie in front of me. I could imagine the aroma and I felt the weight of it on my lap. I saw the little peaks of meringue, golden on their tops, and the crystallike beads of sweat all over the puffy white surface. I saw the heavy gray tin pie plate and the perfectly formed fork ridges on the ledge of the tin. I thought of my mother rolling the piecrust out on waxed paper and the pleasure that she took in preparing the perfect crust. I could see her patching the places that broke as she handled the dough. I could hear her beating the eggs and grating the lemons. . . .

"Suddenly it became clear! I was really seeing my mother's lemon pie. She was the only one I knew who had real tin pie plates. It was she who made such a fuss about the little beads of sweat on the top of the meringue. It came to me in a flash. My mother and I used to make lemon meringue pie on rainy Sunday afternoons. Each Sunday that I had had an urge for lemon meringue pie it had been raining.

"I was amazed at the strong lasting impression that a long-forgotten childhood activity made on my brain. My fear was suddenly gone. I had discovered my real feelings. It was out in the open and I no longer felt fear. There was no more threat to my feelings of confidence. The next Sunday it rained, after my movie, I went to a very nice restaurant. I laughed to myself about the terror that I was permitting myself to build about something that was a very happy memory, cued by rain. I had no trouble resisting lemon pie after that day, although rainy Sundays still remind me of mom and her real tin pie plates."

Margot's experience is not an unusual one. We are taught the eating patterns that we follow and our food preferences. If you experience a special desire for a particular food, analyze it to see if you can develop some insight about the *why* of it. Is it cued by a situation that unlocks your treasure of memories, or is it a real desire for the food itself? If you really crave a particular food, eat it at an appropriate meal. Don't ignore the feelings you have or pretend that it isn't happening. Guard against feeling deprived. Feeling deprived is an uncomfortable feeling. Feelings of deprivation lead to all kinds of unusual behavior. People who don't feel that they are loved enough never grow up to become emotional adults. People who feel that they are deprived of anything rebel in some way. Feeling deprived of foods you crave will distort your perspective until you overeat and binge on the food that you could have enjoyed at an appropriate time and in proper amount.

Use *behavior observation* to search deeper into your real reason for yearning for a particular food. You will enjoy discovery and you will then realize that you are in control. *Know thyself.* And, once again, if you are going to eat, make it worth your while. Eat deliberately or exercise the privilege of deciding *not* to eat. Make decisions. You are the master!

SUMMARY

You have now arrived at a point in your training when you may expect to take responsibility for handling the food in your life. You have the tools. Your confidence is growing with each day of success. Your progress is an outgrowth of your increasing self-respect.

You may expect your weight to fluctuate. You may expect urges for particular food from time to time. You may expect to overeat occasionally. You may also expect days when you have no appetite at all. All of these variations are normal with almost everybody. Eating is one of man's primary drives. Your attitudes about food will change as you control eating. Do not panic when you find yourself daydreaming of eggs Benedict or of cherries jubilee, or when you discover that you gained two pounds during the holidays.

Losing weight has many facets. There will be days when the most carefully planned meals will not result in weight loss. Learn to take these differences in your stride. Accept the fact that food management doesn't just happen! It evolves. It develops. You are the *master!*

Commit yourself by signing the following contract.

Remember that this is a point of honor—a private obligation to yourself:

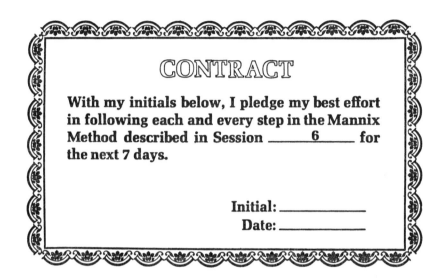

CONTRACT

With my initials below, I pledge my best effort in following each and every step in the Mannix Method described in Session ___6___ for the next 7 days.

Initial: _____

Date: _____

HIGHLIGHTS

A. Go the Distance

1. Move from the mechanics of behavior modification to a psychological support emphasis.
2. Look for your "second wind." It will come just when you need it.
3. Understand fatigue.

B. Cheating

1. Deception is impossible.
2. To eat or not to eat, that is the question!
3. A "swallow" is so fleeting.

C. Plateaus

1. Expect periods of no weight loss.
2. Understand water retention.
3. Concentrate on dimension, not weight.
4. Don't live on your scale.

D. Portion Control

1. Don't use tricks to regulate your portions.
2. Don't weigh food to measure portions.
3. Don't serve food from bowls, family style.
4. Don't linger at the table after meals.
5. Don't do the dishes immediately after eating.

E. Food Journal

Review last week's entries. Under Food/Amount, be aware of food left on your plate.

F. Don't Feel Deprived

1. Understand external cues.
2. Coddle your urges.

G. Weight Chart

1. Weigh yourself and record the weight on your graph.
2. Weigh yourself once a week, no more.

H. Time Allotted for Session 6

One week is allotted for Session 6—as usual.

SESSION 7

FLOW GENTLY

Changing anything, waiting for anything, reaching for anything, requires patience.

It took a long time to acquire your unwanted weight. It will not disappear magically because you are finally facing it. It must change slowly, just as it was acquired. Don't fall prey to impatience now and perhaps try to rush things along by dieting or fasting. You will be setting yourself up for real disappointment later on if you stoop to that at this point. Your goal is to be comfortable with the food around you. Hiding from *fattening* food or skipping meals to lose weight will nurture your fear of food. It will ultimately keep you stuck with fat thinking. As you become thin, you will think fat and you will perpetuate your struggle with eating.

It is very important for you to be proud of your success so far and to practice your new skills with each and every encounter with food.

In a sense, you are now doing a kind of postgraduate work, where the fundamentals are established and training regulations are less demanding. You are now responsible for continuing your own education. You will slowly eliminate many of the training rigors that brought you this far. You are able to shoulder responsibility. It has been serious business to learn "basics" devoid of secrets and hidden magic. You have begun to modify one of your most established behaviors. You had been practicing your eating behavior for all of the years of your life. In just six short weeks you have learned new approaches to eating. You realize success. You are ready for graduate work.

The basic grammar and structure of this new language are established, and you are ready to speak the language with fluency and to think with your newly acquired vocabulary.

You must incorporate your new eating behavior into the automatic flow of daily living. Make sure that your attitude is one of acceptance and that your real goals are always in mind. Add to your strengths each day until you are a thin-thinking, marvelous you.

It takes practice! Practice your new eating skills and flex your new attitude. Don't live on the scale. Pounds lost are not as important as the integration of new eating behaviors. Rigid weight goals and a preoccupation with the loss of weight in pounds will lead to what is called "cognitive claustrophobia." It will increase the temptation to overeat and will perpetuate the fear of food. Don't trap yourself ever again! Keep your goals behavior oriented. Reward yourself frequently to help you to think thin. Think thin and never ever again allow your behavior to master you. You and you only are in the driver's seat. You are in control!

Face one day at a time. Succeed today, and when you retire tonight, add another "win" to your mounting successes. Face tomorrow with the support of yesterday's triumph. You will soon acquire the momentum and the strength of habit. You are fully aware of the tenacity of established habit! Use that knowledge now!

IN RETROSPECT

You have reached the halfway mark. You have effected your most trying adjustments and have begun to recognize your true capabilities. The remainder of the Mannix Method represents a refinement of your new skills. Let's review the tools that you are now ready to polish.

Tapered Eating (Energy/Demand)

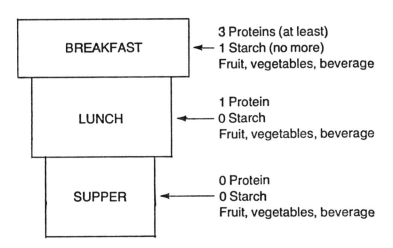

3 Proteins (at least)
BREAKFAST ← 1 Starch (no more)
Fruit, vegetables, beverage

1 Protein
LUNCH ← 0 Starch
Fruit, vegetables, beverage

0 Protein
SUPPER ← 0 Starch
Fruit, vegetables, beverage

No food for at least four hours before retiring.
Include vegetables, fruit, and beverages with an eye to calories.

THE TEN COMMANDMENTS: BEHAVIOR RULES

1. Eat energy/demand Tapered style.
2. Write *before* you eat.
3. Eat only at appropriate places.
4. Eat only. Do nothing else.
5. Enjoy thirty minutes for each meal (pace yourself). Use appestat control.
6. Replace your fork after every bite. Take small bites. Chew well.
7. Take two intermissions, relax for one minute.
8. Eat deliberately—no snacks, meals only.
9. Leave two bites on every plate. Don't run out of food.
10. Delay starting to eat for one minute.

If you have tried any other behavior techniques with success, add them to your bag of skills. Keep using changed daily routines if they are useful.

If you feel hungry at night after dinner, find some absorbing activity to hold your attention until the feeling passes. A walk after dinner helps to establish new routines. Physical exertion decreases hunger, so walk after supper to erase the desire for more food. A bath will always minimize your desire for food. Write a letter to someone who would love to hear from you. Drink a cup of hot decaffeinated coffee or herbal tea to take the edge off. Use any diversion to keep you from slipping back into the old bad habit of eating at inappropriate times.

Use this seventh week to really establish new behavior skills. This is the last week for rigid control. The next session will introduce flexibility in your regimen. The session after that, you will eliminate your Food Journal. Steady yourself now for the next push.

Conditions and procedures will be less demanding now. However, your attention and commitment should be as keen as ever. Demands may diminish, but the need for precision is ever present. You are changing your behavior. To do that, to establish dependable behavior, you must practice, practice, practice.

The Mannix Method is designed to serve you, in your thin state, for the rest of your life. You started swimming upstream by insisting on certain methods for handling food and precise times for eating. As you swim with the tide now and those methods are incorporated, they require less active determination and they are easily implemented. You have more time now for facing life's other demands.

In the past, mood prompted food. Now that you have established your new skills, keep your new eating behavior as a top priority. Your health, after all, is your most valuable possession.

It just takes practice. The twelve weeks assigned to the Method are enough time for you to feel thinner than you have ever felt before. More importantly, you have developed a new attitude about food and about eating. Your new attitude is the key to staying thin. You will stay thin because you think thin. Work on the "thinking"—work on thinking thin. It will seem to happen automatically, but don't stand in your own way. This is old stuff to you now, but dedicate yourself to trying harder. That's how new attitudes take root and grow. Practice makes perfect! Do it again and again. Don't just wish for it—psych yourself into viewing food differently. Keep practicing your skill at each and every meal, one day at a time. Make today a success! Today is all you have, so do it well!

REWARDS

We have previously discussed the importance of rewarding yourself at frequent intervals during your experience with the Mannix Method as your pounds disappear. Let's analyze the reward system and its importance in our lives.

Unfortunately, we have been trained to criticize ourselves for the smallest and the most insignificant errors in judgment, and for the slightest indiscretions. We are taught as youngsters to suppress our feelings and to "act" older, or more responsibly, or more respectfully. We are instructed to be on guard at all times so that our manners are acceptable. In addition to being taught society's code of behavior, we are taught to punish ourselves, should we happen to violate any of those codes. In effect, we are taught self-criticism, guilt, and rejection. We then strive for acceptance and for recognition. Yet there are few rewards to help to motivate us. We all like recognition for a job well done. Instead we tend to criticize ourselves when we really need a pat on the back and some encouragement. A strange dilemma. Our culture feels free to punish and reluctant to reward.

Your rewards should not be just the pounds you have lost. That's a rather negative guidance system. Excess poundage represents something amiss in your life. Reward for lost fat is still playing the "fat" game. You have undoubtedly lost weight before, so losing weight doesn't make you a thin thinker. Attitudes must change with your body size.

Reward yourself every day that you stay on the Mannix Method. It may be just enough to wink at yourself in the mirror at night when you are brushing your teeth. A little recognition. A sign of approval. We all thrive on praise. We enjoy it too infrequently. It takes so little to reward yourself. A peaceful thought of pride as you lie in bed before sleep will top off a successful day. Recognize that you, that person who is you, made your day a success.

Each week completed successfully can clock the time for

significant personal reward. How about a massage each Monday as a reward for respecting yourself? The money that you save by eliminating protein from your evening meals should pay for a massage. Weekly rewards might be anything that delights you. Is it a manicure, a pedicure, a symphony, a stage play, horseback riding, a Sunday excursion? Do something for yourself. Plan something that you enjoy each week to reward yourself for eating to improve your health.

You may choose to reward yourself for significant weight-loss goals. If you work through plateaus, through those frustrating weight plateaus, reward yourself. Celebrate. Take a day off from work, or buy some new flattering clothing and have a party to burn all of your fat clothes. How about some new jewelry if you like jewelry; or take a weekend jaunt. Plan something special.

Reward yourself for extending the length of your walk. Make a list of your favorite activities and treats. Then match your progress points with those rewards. Be generous to yourself. Other people won't praise you—they are too involved with themselves . . . and they *should* be. Praise yourself. You are really the only one who knows how well you have been doing.

One of my clients tells this interesting story:

"As suggested, I began looking at myself in the mirror every morning after my shower. I was looking for the real me to emerge from under a covering of fat and skin that I somehow felt was not mine.

"After a week or so of watching my body for change, I began to comment out loud to my mirror image. It started with a small phrase like 'Not bad at all, old friend,' and after a while that small comment turned into some very helpful counseling.

"I not only commented on my body changes—which, by the way, were noticeably apparent almost each day; I began to say some words of praise to the me that I saw. I didn't do it purposely at first. I had no intention of conversing with myself. But by talking to my mirror image, the me that I stopped to look at, I was able to give that 'me' some praise and some honest advice.

"It was terrific. I came away from those talks every morning like a tiger. I could conquer the world! I learned to look myself right in the eye and to thank myself for being kind, and for having so much respect for me. It made me feel so good that I began saying good night to myself as I prepared for bed. I heard about autosuggestion and how to program yourself by repeating positive suggestion to yourself before going to sleep. I heard about it after I began doing it, so that really reaffirmed my belief in my good sense.

"I began saying good night to my image in the mirror. Soon I included a little pat on the back and a thank-you on the days when I was perfectly satisfied with my behavior. Those days increased, and now I enjoy my company both in the morning and in the evening. I go to bed each night bursting with pride and with confidence. I end my meeting with my friend in the mirror by saying, 'I love me unconditionally. I am a beautiful person.'

"I'm very much in touch with my needs now, and probably for the first time in my life. It took that chance meeting with myself one morning in the bathroom to bring it all about. I am comfortable with food and with eating, probably because I am more comfortable with me. I discovered myself."

FLOODING

Flooding is a technique used to affect the decision-making process. Flooding is forcing yourself to image a frightening situation until the anxiety associated with it disappears, or flows away. Flooding is used in combination with imaging to focus the fears of people with phobias. Flooding forces the fearful image to saturate the senses until its power to cause fear is recognized as simply being the fear of being afraid.

For instance, successful work has been done with people with crippling fear of heights. Severe acrophobia can keep people from going to the second story of a house. It prevents sufferers from boarding elevators and airplanes, from traveling on mountains or crossing bridges. In severe cases it even limits the simple everyday household activity of climbing a stepladder to change a light bulb. The fear has been known to be so intense that some people black out when faced with the possibility of performing the dreaded task. With the use of flooding, these phobic people are forced to face thoughts of heights and of falling. They view films and are instructed to imagine every detail of falling for extended periods of time. They eventually have no energy left for being afraid. Their thoughts are then channeled to imaging a safe, nonthreatening sanctuary to replace the fear that they had just experienced. Repeated sessions of flooding and of imaging will hammer away at a phobia until most of the people who are assisted this way can face heights without crippling fear.

The flooding technique works remarkably well with overeating as well. Flooding is designed to saturate the mind with the problem. How perfectly suited it is in a situation where "filling" is the goal and also the problem. In other words, use your imagination to satiate yourself with food. In your mind fill yourself with your favorite food until you are stuffed to the point of nausea.

Flooding is an exercise to provoke and to agitate, and should be followed with a winding-down period that is soothing. A short period of imaging your safe place would be the ideal way to finish an exercise in flooding.

Pick a favorite food. Sit at your dining table. Close your eyes. Begin to imagine eating your favorite food. At first you eat slowly, with control. Imagine enjoying the food, as you remember it. Begin to eat faster, taking oversized pieces that you have trouble fitting into your mouth. See the food smeared around your mouth and probably stuck to your fingers. The faster you eat, the more food you get on you. Food is falling down the front of you into your lap. Picture your stomach swelling as you stuff more and more into your mouth. Your jaws are stretched open, as in a session with the dentist. Your stomach is bloated larger than you ever imagined it could be. The pain overwhelms you. You are beginning to feel nauseated. The food supply does not diminish on your plate even though you have eaten pounds of it. It actually seems to be increasing in quantity. It is all around you. There's no escape!

Open your eyes. Take a deep breath. There really is no mess around you. You aren't covered with food. Your stomach is its normal shape. The experience is over. Move to another room; sit in a comfortable chair or lie down. Quickly go through your relaxation techniques and close your eyes. Begin to image your safe scene, your sanctuary. Notice every detail. The freshness of the air, the sky, the temperature. Feel serenity flowing through your body and your mind. You are safe, you are warm, and you are healthy. The horrible experience with food is in the past. Feel fresh, feel alive, feel clean.

Formulate your own flooding scenes. Include some of the worst sensations that you can imagine. Use the images of insects in food, or the odor of cat food coming up from your favorite dish. Fill yourself beyond your capacity in your imagination. It will disgust you, and it will help to dissuade you from viewing eating as a hobby. Every time you see that particular food again, recall the flooding experience and the images your imagination associated with that food. Soon you will recall those repulsive associations each time that you see your one-time favorite food. This is highly effective aversion conditioning.

FOOD JOURNAL

Review last week's Journal pages. *Circle* all incidents of inappropriate eating. Then *check* back to each incident to recall the details of each situation. In the space following, *list* any incident of inappropriate eating behavior on one side, and the possible alternative behavior that could have eliminated that incident on the other side. For example:

INAPPROPRIATE EATING BEHAVIOR	ALTERNATIVE BEHAVIOR
1. Skipped lunch—nonstop eating at cocktail party	Eat lunch—control snacking
2. Stopped at theater candy stand—indulged	Arrive late—rush to seat
3. _____	_____
4. _____	_____
5. _____	_____
6. _____	_____

Review all negative incidents carefully. Analyze them. Were you in control? There may be times when you made plans to relax guidelines for special occasions. You took liberties, but you did that because you wanted to. Were you the *master?* Were you in control? Indiscriminate eating, when you are out of control, is something that you may no longer permit yourself.

If you did *circle* some inappropriate eating behavior, eating that was not planned when you were not in control, you must dissect that situation with great care. Those violations were undoubtedly uncomfortable and could have been avoided. Understand the ingredients of those situations.

Permitting yourself to lose control of your eating will rekindle your old destructive feelings of guilt. You then open up the door to using food as a stroking tool, to ease bad feelings of guilt. Then meals have to be skipped to do penance for eating, and then, and then, and then—the old trap. Can you risk that for four inches of tasting pleasure that wasn't even pleasurable at the time? *Examine* uncontrolled eating. Is it ever worth the risk? Instinctive memory records every action and reaction and stores the information for the next time. Each time that you ignore your instinct and reinforce uncontrolled behavior intermittently, you rebuild old habit patterns. They will quietly but *absolutely* reverse the progress that you have made thus far. Can you risk it?

Next week will be the last week for the Food Journal. Devote extra effort to the Journal for the last fourteen days. There is good reason for accuracy with the Journal as you near the end. Your last impression of anything is a lasting memory. Leaving your Journal on a positive note will keep the impressions of it in your memory and will influence your eating behavior forever. Long after keeping records of everything you eat, you will record your food intake in your mind as though you were still using your Journal. Careless record keeping assures weak impressions for later support. These next fourteen days will be most important in your regime. Review all behavior techniques. Increase your effort to record everything and to record it accurately in your Journal. Don't allow yourself to be casual when keeping your records.

PEOPLE WATCHING

Observing people eating in a restaurant is a fascinating experience. People watching can capture your fancy and stay with you.

Keep in mind that anyone whom you observe is on good behavior because she/he is in a public place.

Almost without exception, overweight people eat with more intensity and with more tension than do normal-weight people. You may have noticed, too, that the food selected by overweight people was heavier and usually in combination. There was probably gravy on the potatoes, catsup on the meat, or sauces on other foods.

The obese individual in a restaurant eating a salad is a sight to behold! It is a revelation to study that person. There is usually incredible tension. Fat people on diets get angrier with each bite of food. Very often a large dessert makes up for the sacrifice of the previous dishes. The normal-weight person, on the other hand, usually chooses lighter foods and is less absorbed in eating. Frequent delays during eating are commonplace, and there is usually food left untouched on the plate.

Eating time is significantly different. Fat people may very well finish eating before others have even begun.

When you people watch in restaurants, compare yourself with the people whom you watch. Do you see yourself? Would you like to make some changes?

SUMMARY

You will complete Basic Training this week. You will then depend, and with confidence, on your new eating skills to be completely yours and to give you the security of knowing that you are in control. You are the master of what you do and when you do it. These next few weeks will completely shape your attitudes about food. You will find yourself responding to your improved health by choosing light, delicate food to fuel your body in place of fat-producing heavy meats and starches. It may surprise you that your taste in food is changed so drastically and in such a short time. By being tuned in to your physical needs, your body makes your food choices. Instead of seeking taste thrills, you will prefer food that continues to improve your health. Be alert to new ideas for preparing healthier meals. Make every effort to create interesting, appetizing, and nutritious meals. If your family is eating heavy protein meals at suppertime and you have been eating salads, try cooking an elaborate meal that has no protein or starch. Don't make a "diet" meal. The word "diet" itself spoils appetites. Expend a little extra energy on this first effort. If your family enjoys that first meal, the door will be open to repeating the performance. The whole family will be enjoying healthier meals. Capture their imaginations, excite their taste buds, show them the way.

One client relates his attempt to sway the family's dinner tastes:

"My wife and two preteenagers were very cooperative when I started with the Mannix Method. I announced that I was going to change my eating habits once and for all. I wanted to lose weight and never gain it back again. I knew that they had heard those resolutions many times in the past. Although they were very encouraging, I knew that they were being polite and that they didn't really believe me. They had heard that tune before.

"They were helpful, though, and kept sweets and snack foods stashed away out of my sight. We all enjoyed marvelous breakfasts every morning, without television. And Sally, my wife, prepared delicious salads for me for supper.

"Everything went along so well. I was making progress. My desire for junk food was disappearing. I enjoyed the thirty minutes for eating and relaxing three times a day. But I was uncomfortable at the dinner table. I felt like an outsider with a different menu, with food prepared only for me. The family continued to eat the old way, and I saved my portion of whatever they had for dinner for my breakfast the next morning. I couldn't ask Sally and the kids to forgo their usual food on my account, although they would have done that if I had asked. I realized that I needed more than their cooperation. I needed to change their tastes. I wasn't sure how to do that. I knew that if they would give it a chance, eliminating protein and starch from dinner would make them all feel better. But I was not sure how to lead them into the change.

"I then realized that if I wanted them to change their taste in food, I would have to provide the food. I went to the library one Saturday and looked through cookbooks until I found a cookbook that had some real gourmet vegetable recipes. I copied one that seemed easy enough for me to prepare, and yet fancy enough to be terrific, if I didn't muff it.

"I went home and announced that I would prepare dinner that night. I went to the market to buy the ingredients; some were very new to me, like leeks.

"Sally tied an apron around me and I had a ball making my 'gourmet' meal. If I failed, I would be banned from the kitchen, maybe never to return again. I followed that recipe very carefully. The meal was a four-star success. Sally said it was marvelous. There were no complaints from the kids, which meant that they liked it. I must say that it was good, and for the first time in weeks I felt included at dinner.

"The meal was a real success in a much more important way, though. Sally had heard my message, my call for help. She tried having more original meals made with vegetables. The kids even asked that some meals be repeated. But the clincher came when we invited friends over for dinner one night about a month later. Sally cooked dinner and we were all surprised with Sally's version of my original 'test' gourmet meal. Everyone loved it. It was better than mine, of course. I knew then that I had been a complete success."

Bill had the right idea. Practice your new eating skills and change your environment to support you. The formula is simple. Enlist everyone's help by showing the way.

Now that you can depend on your new behavior patterns, work hard to change your attitude about food. Continue to reward yourself for achieving behavior goals, but also reward yourself for mastering attitudes. When you are able to look at chocolate cake or at ice cream or bread or butter with indifference or even with disgust, you have achieved significant attitude goals. Reward yourself for progress! Treat yourself to something very special when you reach those attitude goals. Attitudes are really what you are striving for.

Reward is absolutely necessary in the Mannix Method of establishing dependable behavior. Don't simply plan on finding those rewards when you reach goals—provide them! You will become goal oriented while your behavior and your attitudes become automatic. Recognize your achievement, reward yourself. Pat yourself on the back. Be your own greatest fan whenever you achieve any goal, be it ever so small. You are an expert at feeling guilty and at criticizing yourself. You have ruined many days and nights with guilt and self-reproach. You know how self-punishment works. Use the same apparatus to appreciate yourself. Praise yourself and busy yourself with rewarding yourself. You have an inner voice that judges you. Use that inner voice to praise when you earn that praise. Praise yourself for learning new eating skills. Praise yourself for changing old attitudes. Praise yourself for feeling happy about your life. Praise yourself for being in control. Praise the master. Sing your praises, when you deserve them.

Review your behavior skills as though you have just been introduced to them. Practice at every opportunity. Don't overlook a single technique when you encounter food. In a few weeks, you will be able to relax rigid restrictions on protein at supper if you wish. But be meticulous until it is time to relax restrictions.

Practice attitude changing. Use *imaging* for relaxation and for developing effective coping responses. Change that old path to food whenever pressure builds, by sidetracking to provide time to turn to alternate activities.

Practice *flooding* with your once-favorite foods. You will be amazed how well the exercise works for you with practice. You will then be able to recall the experience whenever you see that favorite food again. You may even find that it will affect other foods similar in texture and in taste. You have everything to gain by trying all of these techniques. They have been proved effective. They will help you to develop different attitudes about food.

HIGHLIGHTS

A. *Beginning Advanced Work*

1. Practice basic skills. Structure.
2. Incorporate them to become automatic.
3. Think thin.
4. Succeed one day at a time.
5. Make today's success tomorrow's *habit.*

Commit yourself by signing the following contract.

Remember that this is a point of honor—a private obligation to yourself:

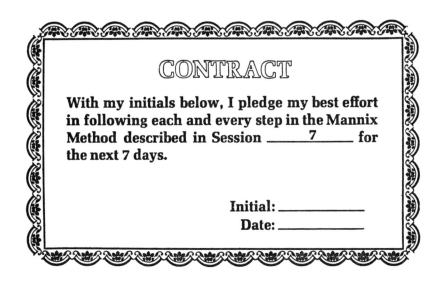

CONTRACT

With my initials below, I pledge my best effort in following each and every step in the Mannix Method described in Session _____7_____ for the next 7 days.

Initial: _____
Date: _____

B. Review Learned Techniques—The Ten Commandments

1. Eat energy/demand Tapered style
2. Write *before* you eat.
3. Eat only at appropriate places.
4. Eat only. Do nothing else.
5. Enjoy thirty minutes for each meal (pace yourself).
6. Replace your fork. Take small bites. Chew well.
7. Take two intermissions, relax for one minute.
8. Eat deliberately—no snacks.
9. Leave two bites. Don't run out of food.
10. Delay starting to eat for one minute.

C. Alternative Activities

1. *Walk* after your dinner.
2. *Bathe* or *shower* in lieu of eating.
3. *Pause* with decaffeinated coffee or tea.

D. Practice to Make Perfect

    1. Practice making changes.
    2. Follow the Mannix Method for twelve weeks.
    3. Succeed just for today.

E. Rewards

    1. Reward yourself *often.*
    2. *Reward* yourself for changing behavior.
    3. *Reward* yourself for new attitudes.
    4. *Reward* yourself without fail.
    5. *Reward* yourself to mark levels of achievement.
    6. *Reward* yourself generously. YOU are the most important
       person in your world.

F. Flooding

    1. Imagine a frightening scene to dissipate anxiety.
    2. Relax after your anxious scene.
    3. Create your "favorite" food in imagination.
    4. Imagine eating, stuffing, gorging—disgusting.
    5. Recall repulsive images to change behavior.

G. Food Journal

    1. Review this week's pages.
    2. *Circle* incidents of negative eating.
    3. Analyze and understand incidents of uncontrolled eating.
    4. Correct intermittent reinforcement.
    5. Anticipate fourteen more days with your Food Journal.

H. Weight Chart

    1. Weigh yourself. Record weight on graph.
    2. Understand the plateaus.

I. Time Allotment

One week for Session 7, as usual.

SESSION 8

PLOT YOUR COURSE

You have mastered all of the techniques that you have learned and that you have practiced so diligently. You are the proud owner of many good, dependable skills. You are ready to move on to new tasks.

The world is a great big wonderful place, full of food. It was relatively easy to control your environment at home or in those familiar places outside of your home space. You must now learn to be comfortable with exposure. You must become comfortable with a variety of food situations. If you anticipate exposure and you have workable plans for coping so that you may control your eating behavior, you will be prepared at any time, in any place, for any situation. You must anticipate situations that involve food. It also helps to research anticipated food situations so that you are not taken by surprise with food encounters. The more you know about any situation, the better you will be equipped to handle it. Do some homework and be prepared. Know yourself and then understand the situation.

Reference is frequently made to the deadly outcomes of surprise attack. Phrases like "gunned down from behind," "stabbed in the back," "caught off guard," "found napping," are familiar to all of us, and they imply a lack of preparation in situations that would have been safe if the victim had anticipated a few of the realities of the world about him. The idea of being victim instead of victor usually implies that a little homework, research, preparation, anticipation, or realistic appraisal might have changed the course of events.

So cover all of the bases in advance. Know the territory before you travel. Don't risk being overwhelmed and then defeated. Anticipate. Plan Ahead. Plot your course. Then forget about it until encounter time.

You have a bag of tools for controlling your encounters with food. Use your skills or you will lose those skills. Keep your tools handy and sharp, and your skills working for you.

One client tells a story about how she felt when her flying instructor got out of the plane and told her to take over alone—to solo:

"I was petrified. I wanted to call him back, but I had no voice. For the first time in my life, I was truly afraid. I was not so much afraid of flying the plane alone; I was more afraid of the trying. I managed to get the plane into the air, and then I wanted to fly all afternoon. I wanted to fly forever."

It is time for you to solo. You have the ability and you have the tools. All you have to do is overcome your hesitation to go.

ANTICIPATE—PLAN AHEAD

Anticipate those old familiar eating situations when you reinforced inappropriate behavior over and over, and then over again. The following may be some obvious recurring hurdles that need your attention. Let's review cues, to establish new cues.

The Theater

If you are accustomed to eating candy or munching popcorn when you attend the theater, you will associate eating with the theater. The theater will act as an external cue to eating. In Session 2, you worked on eliminating external cues to eating. Handle the theater just the way that you handled all of the other external cues. First, *anticipate*. If you always ate in the theater, expect to be cued by the theater. You may count on that before you get there. Now, plan to alter your response to that external cue for eating. *Analyze* the situation logically. Make sure that you are well fed and that you have not rushed through your last scheduled meal to get to the theater on time. Next, *plan* to change one or more of your usual behaviors when you get to the theater. For instance, if you usually go to the theater early and then have extra time to linger around the snack stand, *plan* to arrive at the theater only minutes before the show starts. Go directly to a seat. Select a seat in an area of the theater that is different from your usual. Make changes to weaken cues. Select a seat in the middle of a row so that you have difficulty getting to the aisle and then to the snack stand. Bring a cinnamon stick or some cloves with you to freshen your breath during the show. Eating in the theater may be a result of being inactive and of having a dry mouth. Analyze, anticipate, and come prepared.

Club Meetings

Coffee and dessert gatherings will cue you to eat for sure. Plan to eat nothing for the next few times you go to meetings. Before you go to the next meeting, try to remember what foods were served at the previous meeting. Was it store-bought cookies, greasy doughnuts, gloppy cakes, pastries? Would you really miss not eating them? Think of how much better you will feel after your meeting if you do not eat those unnecessary fat carriers. Satisfy your eating needs before you go and then plan to abstain from eating at the meeting. Don't pledge your life away, just plan to abstain for one meeting—the next one. Don't anticipate never eating at any meeting ever again. Make a separate decision about each meeting right before that meeting.

As you plan for each eating recurrence at familiar events and places, write a balance sheet. Before each occasion, decide on your priorities and examine your investment and your anticipated return on that investment. Do you consider the momentary taste of doughnuts or cookies a sufficient return for weight gain, loss of control, and poor health? Make your plan in advance based on your balance sheet, and then go about your business. It will be simple to make a thoughtful contract with yourself for each occasion and then to honor that bargain.

Parties

Celebrations try our souls. Celebrations encourage abandon, a release from rules and from regulations. The antidote is better planning and realistic appraisal of yourself and the anticipated celebration. Make a balance sheet to establish your priorities and to understand your strengths and your weaknesses. Research the occasion to understand what you will be confronted with. If you can, call your hostess or host to ask about the food to be served. You can usually get this information without really having to ask for it directly. Call on the day of the party to check on the time that you are expected to arrive and in casual conversation about the party, gather some food details. Take them to the drawing board, so to speak. Put the specifics on your balance sheet and plot your eating behavior. Don't be caught off guard.

No matter what the occasion, follow your Tapered Eating. Begin each day with a breakfast of at least three proteins. It may be to your advantage to select lighter proteins so that you may bank some of the calories for the party later that day. Do not skip lunch. Consider having two proteins at lunch so that you are reinforced against hunger at the party. If your blood sugar is high when you get to the party, you will not feel like eating too much. You will not be battling hunger and you will be the master of all you survey. Succeed at one party, and you will succeed at one party after that and one party after that. If someone were to give you a basket of onions to peel, the only way to do them all is to peel one onion at a time. Succeed once, then once again and you will enjoy nothing but success. One success will break the habit of overeating at parties. After your first success, you may look forward to continued control, to continued success. Success succeeds. You will feel marvelous and you will have enjoyed the party for more than its supply of food. Parties will take on a new dimension for you. There is a dimension beyond food that you never knew before.

First, make a list of all the foods that you may expect to encounter. Then plan on the fare that suits you best. If you have not been able to get information about the menu ahead of time, make a tentative map of the territory. Look ahead to salad and to vegetables, omitting potatoes, rolls, and other starches. Remind yourself that you may have any of those other things the next morning for your breakfast. In fact, make plans then and there for your breakfast so that you won't have any possible feeling of deprivation.

Inventory all of your techniques. Match each technique with an anticipated hurdle on a balance sheet. Decide which of the anticipated obstacles can be handled simply with your usual guidelines (sitting down, designating eating places, pacing, pausing, etc.). Anytime that you are able to control an eating situation with one of your usual reliable eating techniques, you benefit in two ways. First, you have the opportunity to abolish thoughtless inappropriate eating once again; and second, you reinforce the technique to make it more dependable. The technique will eventually become automatic behavior.

When your good eating behavior becomes automatic or "second nature," food encounters will be reduced from giants to dwarfs.

The thirty-minute time allotment for meals should be easiest at a party. That's a thirty-minute minimum, of course.

The rule for deliberate eating must always be used in party situations. At any party, if you decide to eat hors d'oeuvres, for instance, eat them deliberately. Select a reasonable portion and a designated eating place, and make it worth your while. Make eating important. Or exercise your option to choose not to eat at all.

Always leave two bites. This is a very easy guideline at a party. Leave two bites on every plate including your hors d'oeuvres plate. Leave two sips of wine in your glass and two sips of coffee in your coffee cup. Leaving something behind becomes a very important tool when you are surrounded by food and drink in abundance. It seems to keep you from being buried in food. It keeps you from nonstop eating. You then know before you start that you will stop. You establish limits. You release yourself from food captivity.

Delay starting for one minute. Apply this rule to every item on the menu, including hors d'oeuvres and finger foods. Your sense of emergency about eating will be relaxed, and you will give yourself the time to mobilize your eating skills.

To assist yourself to eat *deliberately* and slowly, *never talk with food in hand.* Replace any food or any utensil on the plate when you start to talk. Resume eating when you have stopped talking. It is a simple rule of behavior that also makes you a good listener.

You may control most eating at parties and at food celebrations merely by applying your usual rules of eating behavior. The balance sheet will help you to plan ahead. For example, deciding not to eat anything with your fingers may eliminate many pickup foods that are not worth your weight.

Analyze, anticipate, plan, plot your course, and then face each situation prepared. You will control every food encounter with confidence. Face one situation at a time, use a little effort to plan ahead, and then enjoy yourself. Plan to join the fun. Reward yourself for each party well done. Treat yourself to a chic new outfit for the next party. You have earned it.

Holiday Procedures

Holidays are special times in people's lives. They are usually family times. Food is usually a main attraction on most holidays. Thanksgiving, Christmas, Easter. Family and friends together. Holidays are official days to pause and to take it easy. Enjoy the holiday meal with everybody else. Use your usual eating guidelines. Don't be surprised, however, if you find yourself eating far less than you ever did before. What a great feeling of victory! Then reward yourself.

REASSOCIATE

In theaters, at meetings, at parties, and on holidays you face recurring situations that you associate with eating. Inherent in those situations is the suggestion to overeat. Something in your subconscious mind prods you. You need to disassociate those situations from overeating. You may have the feeling that something is missing. The next time you face one of those situations, your task will be to understand the gap in your association. You must understand that if you do not eat, nothing is really missing.

Eliminate the confusion in your memory bank. No mixed signals. Establish new associations so that you don't feel that something is not complete—reassociate. Or, close it off and wrap it up. Follow your plan to be very aware of all external cues to eating inappropriately. Your new control will weaken those old cues. New behavior patterns will dominate so that you will be cued to eat in moderation for the better life.

Expect to alter some situations with one exposure. Others will be more tenacious. They will all fall into line eventually, if you work at it. It is absolutely necessary to handle recurrences deliberately and with definite plan. There will be but a few troublesome stubborn associations that will be managed if you understand them. Analyze the association, understand yourself, and have confidence.

You are growing strong and more comfortable with change. Plan some old familiar routines. Go to a party or give a party. Attend the theater or a concert or a sporting event. Take a drive with several coffee stops. Go to the park or to the beach. Join friends who ate with you. Go to a fair. Spend a lazy day in bed. Stay up late into the night. Try to do everything that you once associated with eating. Reprogram yourself with new appropriate cues. Reassociate. It will pay large dividends. The time that you devote to retraining now is but a short moment when compared to the rest of your life.

Make this job your top priority. In a mere five weeks, you will have completed your training. Only five weeks. A short time for so much benefit. Expend the effort now for the most good. Reap enormous benefits later. Identify inappropriate eating cues as you confront each situation. Force hidden cues into the open.

Anticipate, plan, and then forget about it, knowing that you are prepared. Always reward yourself for a job well done. You will be in control and in beautiful shape for next season's fashions.

ANOTHER LOOK AT DINNER

Let's take another look at completely excluding protein at your supper meal. By now, and certainly when you have completed the Mannix Method, your food needs will have changed drastically. Suppers without protein will be very satisfying and will meet your needs. If you have been conscientious about eliminating protein and have not intermittently reinforced your old habits, you are now ready to tailor your new eating patterns to fit your life-style. You have undoubtedly modified many of your attitudes about eating. Feeling deprived should be a thing of the past.

You will probably find that your first protein-filled evening meal will prove disappointing. You are no longer accustomed to heavy food. You may feel rather uncomfortable. Chances are that you won't sleep as well as you have become used to. You may toss and turn and dream about distressing things. You will awaken tired and without your usual appetite for breakfast. It hardly seems worth your trouble.

Whether or not protein for supper sits well with you, heavier meals at night may be unavoidable and may sometimes be necessary.

A celebration dinner at a special restaurant may be such an appropriate time to include fish or meat in your meal. It is far better for you to enjoy yourself than to feel deprived, punished, and separate. Don't ever put yourself into the position of feeling as though you are dieting. You are definitely not dieting. You are free to eat anything you want. You merely control the *how* and the *when*. If protein for your evening meal seems appropriate, you have developed the skills to handle that change in your routine. Remember, *anticipate* and then *plan* to handle the situation before you get there. *Implement* your plan without any last-minute improvisation.

Anticipate that at dinner next Saturday night you may expect to find alcohol, special breads, enticing appetizers, creative entrees, potatoes, starches, overdressed salads, vegetables, desserts, and coffee. You may further *anticipate* that eating will be leisurely, the conversation interesting, and the service slow. Realizing all of those facts, make a *plan* to fit the whole situation. Identify and weigh the importance of each separate influence. Write another balance sheet to anticipate your decisions about food. If you decide that you will have a drink or perhaps two, then you may want to bank calories by passing up the bread. It may make good sense to plan on skipping the appetizer so that you may really enjoy the entree. Or plan on the appetizer and the salad for your entree. Control the situation so that you may enjoy the best that the restaurant has to offer without consuming unexciting calories and then finding yourself painfully overfed. Skip the potatoes or the pasta—or if they are especially good, take them home for your breakfast. If there is a special dessert, *plan* to have it—if you are not too stuffed at the end of your meal. If you find yourself too full to fit the dessert in, ask to have it wrapped and then take it home for your breakfast. Don't ever allow yourself to eat indiscriminately again. You now belong to the world of normal eaters. Managing food is always practiced by the people in this world who have no eating problem. Start thinking as a thin person thinks and choose your food with care. Make good investments. Never feel deprived. Think thin. Feel thin.

Implement your plan to recognize all of the old cues to overeat. Establish new and more rewarding behavior that allows you to enjoy dinners out and special eating occasions. If you *plan* your approach to food, you will enjoy mealtime more and you will never feel guilty the next morning for your overindulgence and your poor control.

Be sure that heavier dinner meals are the exception and not the rule. You may eat protein for dinner once or twice a week without retarding your weight loss or upsetting your new routine. More frequent indulgence may reinforce old eating habits and undermine the strength of your budding new eating patterns. Don't chance it. Listen to your body needs and *anticipate* reactions to protein-laden evening meals. How will you feel after eating a heavy meal at dinner? Is it worth the change? How will you sleep? Will you be energetic in the morning? Evaluate the possible changes. Your body demands for fuel should direct your control over the why and the when of your eating. All you have to do, and without fail, is to manipulate *how* you eat. Trust your body to demand the right food at the right time. Support your body demands with your new skills for handling each food encounter.

Listen to your body needs, choose the most healthful food, and for a while—until you learn instinctively how much fuel your body can handle at any given time—make a point of not eating too much. You are still training your behavior and you are still molding your attitudes. Don't permit yourself to go back to your old eating habits. Keep in mind that food is a kind of investment. *Plan* your investment so that the return is more than the risk.

A socially active and prominent interior decorator tells of having to attend numerous parties and dinners:

"I was very reluctant to begin this program of weight control with you, as you know, because I believed that I had no self-control, or 'willpower' as you refuse to let me call it. I discuss most of my business around food, either at lunch or at dinner. I travel extensively and I am constantly exposed to food, to good food, with no routine for me to fall back on so that I may feel more comfortable. I have never had to diet. I just started putting on weight in the last two years, as I became known better and I was more in demand as a designer. That was the beginning of fabulous dinners and extravagant parties. It soon became apparent to me that I was overindulging. I didn't know what to do about it.

"I knew that I would not be able to diet away the extra pounds that I desperately needed to lose. I tried to resist some of my favorite foods, which made me angry. I always reacted by eating more than I would have if I had not tried to restrict myself.

"I decided to try the Mannix Method because I was so confused and afraid. I frankly did not know where to turn. I knew that I had to develop some new attitudes about eating rather than find ways to limit quantities of food.

"I began by following Tapered Eating. I was able to stick to the promise that I made to myself by remembering that I would re-evaluate the strict application of the style during my eighth week. That did not seem too long to wait.

"I decided that it seemed best to cancel dinners and parties for the first week so that I could get a firm footing and become comfortable with the Tapered style of my meals. I never used to eat breakfast. I always saved myself for the inevitable stuffing in the evening. So the first thing that I had to adjust to was having breakfast. At first it was difficult to wake up early enough to sit down and to actually enjoy eating. I became a little discouraged. But something very unusual happened on the morning of the third day. I woke up before the alarm clock buzzed. I had never awakened early before. But on this day, I found myself lying in bed with my eyes wide open thirty minutes before the alarm was set to go off. I had to get up. I was wide awake and I was simply astounded.

"I walked right into the shower, which was another thing that I don't ever remember doing before. Still in shock, I watched the sun come up as I dried myself. I felt better than I had ever felt before. I didn't know what was causing it but I felt better than I had ever felt before. I felt strong and healthy and *thin*. I couldn't believe it—I was hungry and ready for my breakfast too.

"As I look back now, that seemed to be the beginning of the rest of my life. Things got better from that point on. By the end of that first 'health week,' as I refer to it now, I was in better shape than I could ever remember being. I had lost only a few pounds, so it must have been something else that was making me feel so energetic and so thin. I didn't care what it was, I was in the pink.

"On my usual schedule the following week, I was a bit uncertain about how I would handle all of the food that I knew I would encounter. I was feeling so good, though, my resolve was strong to stick to Tapered Eating. I was determined to give it the time I had contracted for, and what with feeling so marvelous, I knew that it could be done.

"The first encounter was staggering. There was a table with two smaller platforms on it to form steps. Huge wheels of cheese from all over the world were placed from top to bottom and then garnished with orchids flown in from Hawaii that morning. There was another table with a four-foot pyramid of shaved ice, rising out of a bed of tropical shells and iridescent stones. Embedded in the shaved ice were oysters on the half shell, larger than I had ever seen before. There must have been a few hundred oysters in the ice. There was an attendant standing by dressed in a starched white cotton suit with shiny brass buttons, waiting to replace the oysters as they were removed from the ice. Waitresses poured champagne and passed food on trays so that you didn't have to go to the food at the buffet.

"I was so impressed with the display that by the time I got around to remembering my pledge not to eat inappropriately, the idea of eating anything seemed completely out of the question. I was amazed with myself. All of that glorious food and I didn't want any. I couldn't believe it. I even walked over to the cheese display to examine some cheeses from parts of the world that I didn't know made cheese. I almost wanted to want something so I could deny myself, just to test my determination. I found it hard to accept the fact that I wasn't suffering in that land of plenty.

"I remember chuckling to myself and taking a deep breath. I sipped a single glass of champagne and left all of that food behind. I moved through the crowd during the party and I never once thought about eating again that evening.

"When I left the party later that evening and thanked the hostess, I realized I had had more fun at that spectacular party than ever before. I realized I had enjoyed myself so much because I was not busy stuffing my mouth and feeling fat and clumsy. I left the party filled instead with nice memories. I felt stimulated, not stuffed.

"After that first party, all of the other parties were easy to face. After all, if I didn't have to gorge myself that time, why should I anticipate failure any other time? Dinners turned out to be pretty easy too. I had never noticed before that there are always more than enough vegetable dishes at any dinner party to keep anyone happy. I was determined to practice my new Mannix Method for the suggested time.

"At the eighth week I allowed myself to reevaluate my having protein in the evening. I tried it a few times, and now I think that I want to exclude it entirely all of the time. I felt worse for having protein every time I tried it. It made me uncomfortable and spoiled some of my fun.

"I'm not afraid of food situations anymore. I know that all I have to do is be guided by my body cues. It's funny how we fear things that are really not frightening. In the past the fear of not being able to control my eating at parties always drove me to overeating so I could handle the fear. I thank the powers that be that I am rid of that trap."

There is no food situation you find yourself in that you cannot control. Don't be afraid of going out to eat. Don't fear any change in routine. *Anticipate,* make a *plan,* and then don't worry about it until you *implement* your plan. You can't go wrong. Eat deliberately. Don't pick at food or try to sneak food with your old carelessness. It doesn't work. Your body counts every calorie that you take.

Your new skills will shape your attitude with each new food encounter. Trust the Mannix Method. Depend on your ability to handle any situation that involves food. If you want protein in your supper meal, have it. Use all of your eating skills and then trust your body to set the limits.

If you should happen to reach a plateau with your weight loss after reintroducing protein at your evening meal, discontinue the late protein immediately. It is very important that you maintain your weight-loss momentum. Your metabolism is accustomed to utilizing your fat at a steady pace. The extra protein may alter that process. So if your weight loss stops with the introduction of evening protein, discontinue it. Postpone protein to another time when your body chemistry is better able to handle it, or when you have reached the physical thin you to match your mental new thinness.

Above all, be patient. Subtle changes will be made from here to the end of the program. Remember, it is not like stopping a locomotive. The Mannix Method is a process, not an event. It will shape your way of life. Adjusting your eating techniques and the continuing shaping of your attitudes about food are your goals right now. Hold steady to your course. Do not try to go faster than the Mannix Method takes you.

Reward yourself each and every time you demonstrate your mastery in any eating situation. Were you in control? Did you rearrange the environment to meet your needs? Were you the Victor, not the Victim? Salute the master and reward yourself immediately. Mark your progress en route to your trim world. If you neglect to reward yourself, you may suffer from a feeling of deprivation. You will not be replacing the old pleasure of food gratification with another kind of pleasure. Make the reward for exercising your control more important than the old reward of eating. You will be avoiding inner conflict and at the same time you will be reinforcing new pleasure. Reward yourself handsomely for each win. Sing your praises, because you are on the final stretch home. Spend some time and some money on yourself. You are the most important person in your world. You are succeeding at being successful. Put all failure behind you with some special prize.

FOOD JOURNAL

Review your Journal.

This is the last week that you will be keeping the Journal. Keep your records accurate and remain thorough for these next few days. Your Journal has been your most valuable tool during your journey. It has shaped your thinking about eating. It has taught you to plan and to be aware of the food in your life. As you continue to use the Journal for this last week, focus on the purpose for recording everything *before* you eat. When you eliminate the Journal, you will want to continue to *anticipate* your meals and to *plan* the proper food for energy demand.

After this week, you won't *write* before you eat. You will *think* before you eat. You will make records in your mind. Maintain the effort you used to write in your Journal so that you may use that effort to *think* before you eat.

It should take you about one week to make the transition to mental recording. Each time you write in your Journal this week, stop to think about what you are doing. Visualize exactly what it is that you are about to put into your mouth. Don't write your entries without thought. Stop. Think. Pause. Think before you write. Prepare yourself to keep mental records.

SUMMARY

At the close of this session, there will be only twenty-eight days left for you to complete the Mannix Method. As you lose weight, you reshape your attitudes about the role of food in your life, and the importance of your health. The Mannix Method is an invitation to good health. It uses the control of eating, with the subsequent weight loss, as the road to good health. If you become healthy in body, you will also become healthy in mind. The state of being healthy will be incompatible with being fat. You are losing your fat as the result of improving your health. In order to gain weight back, you will have to witness the deterioration of your health. It is unlikely that you would sacrifice your wonderful feeling of well-being for four inches of taste thrill.

To insure that your momentum carries you on to your goals, don't miss the advantage of *anticipating* every possible food encounter. Then make a *plan* and *implement* it. Make your plan work. Don't chance being off guard. Use your skill to keep you thin and healthy forever.

Stay in control of your eating even if you don't have control over food. Forget the old diet tricks that you used to use to repent for inappropriate eating. Remember fasting the day after or the day before a dinner party? Remember being your own whipping boy? Instead, exercise control over eating. There is no such thing as "cheating." There is no need for deprivation. Just stay in control. Follow Tapered Eating for meals. Eat to get thin. Eat to stay healthy.

Refrain from running to your scale to monitor the damage that was done after you lost control. Merely get right back to Tapered Eating and select foods that are a little lighter and more delicate. Use your bag of skills to make sure that you never feel hungry or deprived. Never feel guilty about enjoying yourself. Never feel defeated for breaking your usual routine. Blame, guilt, feelings of deprivation, self-pity, and defeat are the ghosts of your past. Put them behind you forever with your old fat body.

Success requires some new responsibilities, some new expectations, new obligations. The obligation is to you—that most important person. You must believe in yourself. You must like yourself. You must be kind to yourself. You must believe in success to make success dependable.

HIGHLIGHTS

A. Anticipate, Plan, Implement

Recurring situations: Develop new associations. Depend on new skills. Anticipate the hurdles. Plan on changes. Put your plan to work. Implement the plan.

1. The Theater: Alter your old behavior chains. Sit in a different place; arrive late; bring cloves or cinnamon to munch.
2. Meetings: Eat before you go. Establish priorities. Know the obstacles to find a solution. Handle one meeting at a time.
3. Parties: Do some research. Anticipate the pitfalls. Consult your balance sheet. Succeed at the first party to win them all.

Commit yourself by signing the following contract.

Remember that this is a point of honor—a private obligation to yourself:

CONTRACT

With my initials below, I pledge my best effort in following each and every step in the Mannix Method described in Session ____8____ for the next 7 days.

Initial: _____

Date: _____

4. Holidays: Enjoy family, friends, and food. Use your skills. Never skip meals before the banquet.

B. Reassociate

1. Replace inappropriate eating cues—disassociate.
2. Implement your plan exactly. Control will overcome old cues. Old associations will be closed.
3. Force old associations to close them out.
4. *Anticipate; plan;* then forget about it until encounter time.
5. Reward success.

C. Review Your Evening Meal

1. Tailor new eating habits to fit your life-style.
2. Include protein when appropriate.
3. Feel victorious. You are not on a diet.
4. Eat anything you want. Control *how* and *when.*

5. Plan ahead to avoid last-minute variations.
6. Write a balance sheet. Eliminate no-value foods.
7. Include dinner protein as the exception, not the rule.
8. Recognize the change in body chemistry with the change in food.
9. Reward success.

D. Food Journal

1. Review.
2. Analyze your purpose.
3. Think before you write.
4. Think before you eat.

E. Weight Chart

1. Weigh yourself and graph your weight.
2. Enjoy your success.

F. Time for Session 8

One week, as usual. Use it all.

SESSION 9

CELEBRATE

Aren't you amazed and thrilled with your progress so far? It is all the result of *wanting*. It is the result of wanting to change your life-style, so that the new person who is emerging can be realized. The new *you* is in the process of becoming. You were always there waiting to be freed.

Reward yourself this week with something that will make you happy. Have you been dreaming of some faraway place? Why not go there? Plan something very special and make those plans right now. You have worked diligently on this program, and you have altered some deeply entrenched habit patterns that seemed to be totally inflexible. You found the courage to change. You climbed many mountains, you fought many battles. You persevered. Now celebrate! Learn to be generous with yourself. You probably never permitted yourself to be good to yourself before. Weren't you eager to do for others and not do for yourself? With this alteration of your body dimensions, you have also altered your view of yourself. Guilt, self-reproach, and blame are no longer in your vocabulary, nor in your thoughts. You are your closest admirer, worthy—in fact deserving—of the good things in life. Reward yourself for accomplishment. Treat yourself every now and then just for being.

You may now start to relax some of the rules and the regulations of your routine so that you may be free to make choices. It is important to finish off each level of your growth so that you may start each next level with renewed enthusiasm. Mark each new beginning with something special for yourself. You completed the bargain that you made with yourself; now mark it. Your old pattern of failure is a thing of the past.

We are all so eager to criticize ourselves and so reluctant to praise. We are trained to be embarrassed to praise ourselves. But praise is nourishment for the mind. Don't risk the malnutrition of your life center. Treat yourself. "If you are not good to yourself, *who* are you?" Reward yourself to mark your progress thus far. Could you have done better? Well then, now is the time to try. Regret is a waste of energy and of time. Instead, begin right now to achieve your goal for today. Give you your daily bread! Forget yesterday—all the yesterdays—and even the tomorrows. The time is NOW.

EXERCISE YOUR SKILLS

Assume more responsibility for defining your own choices. Dedicate yourself to living life as a *thin* person, with all of the skills to continue losing weight if you wish. You have the skills to remain *thin* forever. Use those skills. Make those skills a part of all of your eating existence. For instance, always *replace* your fork after each bite of food. Do it automatically, without thinking. Control your portions. *Delay* starting to eat for one minute. Take two *intermissions* during every meal. These simple techniques will keep you free from inner bondage. Respect food and look forward to eating with a feeling of dignity.

Managing food is not punishment, nor is it a form of deprivation. Average people always manage their eating. Practice your management skills so that you stay *healthy* and *thin* for as long as you live. Thinking *thin* is nothing more than just thinking. Use your mind, not your mouth, to manage everything in your day, including food.

Controlling your behavior is merely thinking and planning. Become aware of what you do. Control is just being in charge. Control is just having a design for living. Control is anticipating what comes next. Being in control is simply using your natural endowment to run your life.

You now know the *whys* and the *wherefores* of your eating. You are in control. Losing weight is only *one* of the results of control, and it is perhaps the least important product of your control. Your major triumph is your new ability to stay in control of your eating forever. You will, therefore, stay thin forever. You need never again be obsessed with food, nor be victimized by it. You are free to think of many other things. Welcome to the normal world! Welcome to a world where eating and food are not your total existence.

COPING ALTERNATIVES

It should be obvious by now that much of your eating was a response to frustration and to disappointment. It was used as a coping mechanism, a way of dealing with your emotions. We all need mechanisms for coping with life's trials and tribulations. But we do not need ways of coping that compound our problems and further complicate our already complicated lives. We need to cope to solve problems, not to create more problems.

One client, Janet Kanter, tells of an interesting way of dealing with her drive to eating-to-cope-with-frustration.

"I imagine a voice that urges me to treat myself to food. It's like a devil, an evil person outside of me trying to steer me in the wrong direction, against myself. Whenever he speaks up, I talk back. I ask him *why*. I make him tell me what made him so angry and why he wants to punish me. Our talking back and forth gives me many reasons for my inability to cope with my real problem.

"I know it sounds kind of nutty. I always go someplace to be alone when I play this game, so I can feel free to talk or even to yell. Many times I wind up crying and beating my hands on the pillows, but it always works. I'm always able to redirect that drive to eat. The most incredible thing that has come out of my dialogues is how much I've learned about myself. I almost always discover what it was that motivated me to begin with. It may have been disappointment with myself for not doing as well as I could have in a particular situation during that day, or treating someone in a shabby way, or taking on the problems of the world to my detriment without liking myself first. I then punish myself, or the other me punishes me by pretending that eating will make bad situations better. It never works. I know that now. It only adds another, bigger problem.

"I am also finding that I have these 'talks' less frequently as time goes by. I have developed some insight about what triggers me before things happen and I can then catch myself before I get trapped. The Mannix Method is helping me to live better as well as to live thinner."

Find constructive ways to cope with your life problems. After all, life is but a series of problems that need solution. Find ways of coping that will ease disappointment and at the same time will alleviate frustration. Don't let your shelter become your prison. When you feel good you don't have to punish or hide or escape. You have eliminated the eating-to-cope mechanism that compounded your difficulties.

"I used a technique something like Janet's," reports Jane Whitfield. "Whenever I feel the need to eat when I feel rotten, I go to the bathroom mirror, and I look myself straight in the eye and I say, 'Okay, just what are you trying to do?' I have whole conversations with that other person in the mirror. Sometimes things are said that really startle me. I hear some things that I never knew were in my thoughts. Sometimes I embarrass me. But I work things out this way. It's very easy to deceive yourself when you carry on the debate in your head. It's another situation entirely when you are face to face with yourself and talking out loud. You can't lie. You must tell the truth. The truth has always been that I don't want to punish myself. I love me, and being thin and in control of my own life is more important to me than any mouth full of anything. It all comes out in my talks with myself in the mirror. My life must have no more self-deception."

Tension is inherent in frustration and in anger. Coping with tension permits you to be free to solve life's inevitable problems. Both Janet and Jane released tensions by talking them out with themselves. The psychiatrist's primary function is to help you to ease the by-product of life's frustrations. To cope is to adapt. You make the best out of what is available when you cope comfortably.

There are many tension-releasing activities that you may want to explore in your search for alternate coping methods. In order to face the problems that you need to solve, be they small or large, you must alleviate your tension. Tension blurs your thinking. You will cope with any situation to the best of your ability if you can relax enough to think.

You will be free to discontinue your daily walk next week, if you choose to do that. But this week, try walking a little faster for a shorter distance. Or jog a short distance and walk a short distance. Getting out of breath is a good way to release tension. Runners say that they not only relax their minds when they run, they experience a "high."

Golf is a relaxing and tension-draining activity. Bowling or dancing will also help to relieve tension. Even reading or playing chess relieves tension by refocusing your attention.

The best method there is for relieving tension and avoiding your coping-by-eating practice is imaging along with your body relaxation techniques. You must find ways to relieve the tension caused by life's many frustrations. Live a happier, healthier life by coping with tension so that you may think. Make coping-by-eating so difficult that you will actually force yourself to discover alternate ways to scale life's hurdles.

It is easy to do well when you feel good and are full of confidence, but no one feels bouncy and great all the time. All of life has a rhythm, a series of changes. Try to understand your mood rhythm so that you may anticipate your "downs." And then, when you make your plans, your coping plans, keep an open mind and a closed mouth.

Devise protective eating rules and be prepared with diversions to help you to alter those habitual coping-by-eating episodes. Remember, you may feel bad today and bouncy tomorrow. One of the dependable certainties of life is change. Change is absolute. Find ways to cope to take you through bad times without body damage. Learn to cope with life so that you live better longer.

Keep in mind that no matter how "down" you may feel right now, coping-by-eating will surely make you feel worse. In addition, it will diminish future pleasures. It's a losing syndrome. You can never win when you eat to alleviate frustration. From bite to swallow, there are only four inches. You taste food for no more than thirty seconds and you remember it for less than one minute. That's the most that you can hope for; that is, if you are really eating deliberately and you are concentrating only on food. In every case of eating-to-cope, food enjoyment is a low priority. In fact, it is nonexistent. Coping-by-eating involves food rather incidentally. Eating, ingesting, filling, stuffing. The activity is the purpose. The doing something is the coping mechanism, not the food.

Losing weight was your heart's desire. Forget about food until you are hungry. Cope with disappointment and frustration with your mind, not with your mouth. View food as a requirement for good health and for your emotional well-being. If you anticipate an eating disaster coming your way, *change* your environment, or find a diversion, or just recognize the situation. Enjoy the pleasure of eating control. It will feel good. Feel proud, feel strong, feel lean. Have the confidence to find intelligent solutions to real problems instead of turning your back on this that is your life. Keep your mind off food when it is not appropriate to eat. In addition to the active things that you have been using to consume your attention, there are many small changes you can make to jolt you out of a possible food trance. One of the most effective jolters is perfume. The instant overwhelming fragrance of perfume will take your mind off food long enough for you to think. Your smelling apparatus is connected to your tasting apparatus. The aroma of good food excites the appetite. Saturate your nostrils with the fragrance of perfume and you will redirect your thoughts to physical sensation, where feeling slender and graceful is your preference. Four inches of taste, and then you wear it. Put your mind where your mouth is so that you may use your other senses.

Whenever you feel that you may be losing control—and to err is human—take a d-e-e-p breath, then hold it, hold it for four seconds. Then e-x-h-a-l-e very s-l-o-w-l-y. As you exhale, systematically release all of your muscle tension. Start at the top of your head and move into your relaxation routine. Practice this "releasing" immediately, whenever you feel strained. Relaxing will put you right back in the driver's seat. If d-e-e-p breathing or the tongue pressure technique (Session Four), or both, are not enough to redirect you, reach for the perfume, or take a shower, or a walk, or brush your teeth, or drink a large glass of water. Or combine remedies. Experiment. Find various tricks or combinations of tricks to capture your attention, so that you may alter your path to unnecessary food. If you give yourself a little time to settle down and gather your thoughts and your strength, turning to food to cope with a situation will no longer make sense to you.

The key to coping adequately is to relax your body and to refocus your attention. Then your body will be a pleasure to wear. Your body will be a beautiful place to be, and just the right size for you.

Food Days

There are days in everyone's life when a kind of unrelenting appetite just will not be satisfied. No amount of food seems to appease the need to eat on those strange days.

There is no exact explanation for those unusual days. Don't let those days frighten you. "Food days" are part of most people's experience, and are therefore quite normal. There are some days when your body needs more than the usual amount of sleep, even though you have not changed your usual regime of activity. Your body may need extra fuel on those puzzling food days. Don't worry about it, just handle it to the best of your ability. Divert your attention for assistance. Postpone urges for very damaging foods to an appropriate meal, if you can.

Don't ever skip a meal on those "food days." It is far better to allow yourself unusual food at any of your meals than to devour what you crave in the car or in front of the refrigerator, hoping that the urge to eat will leave after the stuffing. Make it a meal, if it is worth your time and attention. Eat deliberately.

Exercise as much control as you can during those trying days, but don't punish yourself. Recognize some of the limitations of your being and accept the drive as unwanted, annoying, but normal. It happens to most people every once in a while.

Be flexible. Adjust to any unreasonable appetite by providing more food at the correct times. Muster all of your wonderful techniques to weather the storm. This too shall pass. Weather the storm with courage, and without your old attitude of despair. Accept your limitations and imperfections, knowing that perfect behavior is impossible all of the time. This is but a small break in the continuity of your program that may be remedied in a matter of hours. Above all, do not fall prey to that old destructive guilt-and-punishment routine.

EATING ONLY AND ALONE

At the start of the Mannix Method, you were asked not to perform any other activity when you were eating. The reason for that requirement, of course, was so that you could give your undivided attention to the experience of eating. You would then be right there with all of your mind and your senses to experience the signs of feeling full, of feeling satisfied. Another reason for "eating only" was to eliminate the external cueing of the other activity. We are all familiar with the path to the refrigerator from the television set, cued by the commercials on your favorite programs.

By this time in the Mannix Method, you have extinguished all of those external cues for eating. Twenty or thirty minutes are now devoted to each of your meals, depending on whether or not you finish everything in the meal. You experience the taste and the sensation of food. You delay starting to eat each meal for one minute, at least. You take two one-minute intermissions during each meal, to eliminate any sense of emergency about eating and to relax. You are in control. Your control skills are your prized possessions. Keep those skills sharp. They serve you well.

The single most important skill that you have, to stay in control of your eating, is the thirty-minute-per-meal technique. It prevents binge eating and emotional eating. Practice that technique above all else, no matter what you are faced with. Postpone your meal until you can make thirty minutes available. That time allotment will be your port in a storm.

Now that you are a person in control of your eating and your living, you may modify the rigid requirement of eating without any other activity. Eating, as an isolated activity, may have made thirty minutes seem forever. You are now ready, if you wish, to read while you eat.

Reading while eating is permissible if you are able to dissociate the two activities, so that you don't fall prey to external cueing. You must separate the activities in your mind and in your time. How is this done? When you read, have nothing to do with your food. When you eat, have nothing to do with the reading material. It is rather like a good marriage, where things operate together but must remain separate.

The ideal way to do this is, first, sample your food s-l-o-w-l-y for a bite or two in your usual way. Replace the fork on the plate. Then open your book or your magazine over to the side of the plate (newspapers are a little clumsy at first). It is very important that you do not read over your plate. Place the reading material off to the side where you can't see the food. You might try crossing your legs to the side of the table so that you may place your book on your knee. This position forces you to twist to the side to pick up your fork to eat. It is an awkward position for your body, so as soon as you take one mouthful, you are forced to put your fork down to turn again to your reading, away from the table.

Read until you come to a natural break. That place may be halfway down a page or two pages away. Don't stop your reading in the middle of an idea or theme because you have food on your mind. Train yourself to concentrate completely on reading without competing thoughts of food. If you find that reading and eating compete so that you cannot concentrate, give the full amount of time to eating as your only activity. To avoid external cueing, it is extremely important to be able to keep eating as a separate activity in your mind.

However, if you can handle a dual activity, reading with eating can help to slow you down. Thirty minutes for eating when you eat alone can be less demanding of your patience if you are able to perform two separate activities at the same time. Be careful to devote your full attention to each of the activities separately. Read when you read, giving the written word your full attention, and eat when you eat. If you read a newspaper with your meal, use your full attention and both of your hands. Divide your time at the meal, but do not divide your attention.

And remember, do not sacrifice those two marvelous intermissions during your meals. Push yourself away from both the food for body and the food for mind (the reading), for just one minute to assess your degree of fullness. And, of course, you will leave two bites on the plate with every meal. Leaving food on your plate at every meal reminds you, beneath your conscious level at this point, that you have had quite enough to eat. You know now that the amount of food you see is not the amount of food you need to satisfy your hunger. You have eliminated all of the external cueing that used to work to destroy you.

FOOD JOURNAL

Review the pages in your Food Journal for the last time. You are about to discard your training wheels. You are finished with your written record keeping and you must now continue the monitoring with your mind.

If you look forward to putting the Food Journal aside, don't put aside planning for control. You must continue to eat deliberately and thoughtfully. You will never again eat anything that you have not considered deliberately. Make a "mental note" of everything you eat. Know your position at all times, right through every day. Eat *deliberately*, with purpose and a sharp practiced sense of awareness.

Replace your Food Journal with knowledge and with self-confidence. You are trained to handle food on your own, and the further use of the Journal may begin to be a needless crutch. You have the skills to stand straight and strong. You have courage, training, stamina, and self-respect. You know that you are capable of doing what you really want to do. You have made many discoveries during these weeks. You discovered that you were the victim of fear many times, when there was nothing to be afraid of except that very fear.

You are a winner and you can continue to win as long as you take one step at a time and then give it all you have. Give it your undivided application. Put your Food Journal aside for this next meal. Plan the meal and prepare it with your usual concern. Plan and prepare all of the meals following as if you were writing the plans in your head. It's easy.

Be very deliberate, plan slowly, and stay in control. Deliberation, design, purpose, were the goals of Journal keeping. You had to think before you wrote. Now just concentrate on the planning. Don't allow yourself to eat anything that you don't really want, or that you are not hungry for. *Think* before you eat. Put your mind where your mouth is.

Eliminating the Food Journal is a giant step. Guard against the destructive temptation to taste food every once in a while, to eat just a few peanuts if you happen to pass an open jar. Be alert for nasty old habits creeping back, like tasting while cooking, or sipping soft drinks during the day, or finishing some of the children's leftovers. They are all rather innocent, innocuous actions, but they will erode your control, and they will change the shape of your living place.

In fact, try to be more careful for the remaining three weeks on the Mannix Method about *how, when, where,* and *what* you eat than you have ever been before. Practice *not* keeping the Food Journal with the same dedication that you used to keep it. Learn to solo without the Food Journal, keeping records in your head. Eat deliberately, having made your plans with care and purpose. Put your mind where your mouth is.

SUMMARY

Life, in a complicated, overpopulated society, is difficult at best. Stress is no longer reserved for those in high places. We all live with stress every day of our lives. Scholars have named the twentieth century The Age of Anxiety. We are a world of people victimized by technology. The individual may be overlooked for the collective good of society. Individuals are sometimes lost in statistics. Coping skills are absolutely necessary for one's survival. Coping-by-eating is a self-destructive way of dealing with the stress of living. Overeating merely diverts your attention and produces more stress and more problems. Coping-by-eating is just another form of self-deception, an avoidance technique, a destructive form of self-deception. It is a kind of false, temporary shelter that keeps you locked in.

Grow into the maturity of dealing with life's inevitable problems by facing what needs to be done, and then take one step at a time. Recognize your limitations and accept them. Recognize your talents and use them. Accept yourself by respecting yourself. It is estimated that sixty percent of the population of this country is overweight. That statistic represents a staggering amount of poor adjustment. It represents pounds of self-rejection, pounds of needless anxiety.

Change it! Take one task at a time, one step at a time, peel one onion in the basket at a time. Find constructive new ways to cope. Shape your body with self-respect. Control your eating one day at a time. Everyone has the privilege of growing into maturity. Shed your childish, emotional shelters for the privilege of moving on to adult control. Remember, excessive eating is a poor substitute for real emotional satisfaction. Reach for the real thing and you will grow tall instead of fat.

Commit yourself by signing the following contract.

Remember that this is a point of honor—a private obligation to yourself:

CONTRACT

With my initials below, I pledge my best effort in following each and every step in the Mannix Method described in Session ____9____ for the next 7 days.

Initial: _____

Date: _____

HIGHLIGHTS

A. Be Good to Yourself

1. Celebrate your progress.
2. Reward yourself generously.
3. Accept additional responsibility.
4. Practice food management every time you eat:
   a. replace your fork;
   b. avoid standing;
   c. delay beginning;
   d. take two intermissions.
5. Consider food management part of normal living. Everyone uses it.
6. Think to control. Plan to control.
7. Put your mind where your mouth is.

B. Coping Alternatives

1. Avoid eating-to-cope.
2. Understand that life is a series of problems to be solved and resolved. That's what it is all about.
3. Learn to handle frustration:
   a. talk to yourself in a mirror;
   b. try some self-analysis;
   c. use relaxation with deep breathing;
   d. distract your tasting apparatus with perfume odors;
   e. brush your teeth;
   f. write yourself a letter;
   g. drink a glass of water;
   h. take a walk;
   i. bathe or shower to pamper your body.

C. Food Days

1. Accept the fact of unreasonable appetite days.
2. Understand the situation without blaming yourself for losing control. Blame and guilt are things of the past.
3. Use all of your behavior rules.

4. Provide more food at appropriate times. Don't snack.
5. Know that this too shall pass.

D. Eating Only and Alone

1. Experiment with reading if you eat alone.
2. Keep activities separate. Alternate them.
3. Take the usual two intermissions. Do not read or eat during intermissions.
4. Continue to leave two bites on your plate. They remind you that you have had enough to eat.

E. Food Journal

1. Eliminate your Food Journal this week.
2. Make mental notes of everything that you eat.
3. Think before you eat.
4. Eat deliberately. Put your mind where your mouth is.

F. Weight Chart

1. Weigh yourself.
2. Graph your weight on the chart.

G. Time for Session 9

One week, as usual.

SESSION 10

Simple Logic

Boredom breeds obsession. Obsessive thinking produces compulsive behavior. Boredom is therefore the breeding ground for binge eating—for compulsive, unreasonable eating behavior.

Since you have been working with the Mannix Method, you have undoubtedly noticed that on those days on which you are alive and involved with things that you enjoy, thoughts about food are rather infrequent. You may even have found that you had to make a conscious effort to eat your regular meals. You were then easily satiated. Those days were the exact antithesis to the "food days" discussed in the last session.

Eating is sometimes used as a substitute for the real emotional satisfaction that comes with involvement and productivity. Feelings of accomplishment and of pride use the psychic energy that is otherwise diverted to oral satisfaction. Get busy and get "high" on yourself. Food will then fall into its proper perspective. When you permit yourself to fall by the wayside, you seek pleasure in unrewarding pursuits. Look for satisfactions that spark your brain and propel you into the world at your maximum pace.

Boredom breeds obsession because it allows you the time to dwell on thoughts about food. Then, the more you think about food, the more you become obsessed with it. Your obsessive thinking leads to compulsive eating. It all starts with a void in your thinking. Direct your thoughts outward instead of inward, and keep your hours filled with things that give you feelings of satisfaction and reward and relatedness.

It may be necessary to review and then perhaps to change some structural parts of your living pattern to keep your thoughts flowing outward. You have a moral obligation to become free, loving, warm, and positive. Systematically examine your eating history again, now. Your viewpoint is a more objective one at this stage in your training. Boredom, frustration, anger, disappointment, separateness, aloneness, were probably the feelings, better named the culprits, that drove you to cope with your mouth.

Analyze and study your life patterns anew to discover areas that still give you difficulty with control. Identify those areas and develop some insight about them; you may then set about changing parts of them to make your living more rewarding. Remember, in making the change in any chain of behavior, the slightest alteration in the usual order of events (links) may make a great big difference in the product. In Session 3, you remember that you altered a few links in each of your behavior chains. You examined your daily ritual patterns so that useless behavior could be discarded or replaced. The procedure is exactly the same, except that now you must examine whole segments of your way of life that may have become obsolete.

Find the parts of your life that leave you feeling frustrated or bored to death, or trapped and immobilized. When you find those parts of your life, face them honestly and begin to free yourself from immature frustrations. Until the day you die, you can change and discover many of your hidden untapped resources. Life is an unfolding process. Life is discovery. Life is the discovery of self and its development. There are those of us who have chosen to turn from life, to hide from life, and who choose to die each day that they live. They commit a kind of partial daily suicide that uses all of their energy and blinds them to their talents and natural wealth.

Examine your work. Does it challenge you? Does it keep you occupied? Is it satisfying? How can you make it more rewarding?

Examine your leisure-time activities. Are you busy with things that you enjoy doing, with things that give you feelings of contentment? Do you have a dream?

Examine your relationships. Think about your friends, business associates, and relatives. Are you honest about your relationships? Are your friendships simple and satisfying, or are they frustrating and destructive? Simple, uncomplicated affection is a necessary ingredient for living. It is necessary to give love and affection to be healthy.

There is no question that your environment can keep you fat. You have learned to control your eating patterns. You can also control your immediate food environment. Your final step is to flex your total life-style. Analyze the structure of your personal world.

IN CONTROL

"As I began to feel successful controlling my eating," reported Julie Brooks, "I found myself cleaning my closets, relining my dresser drawers, and balancing my checkbook the day I received the statement. One Saturday afternoon, I realized that I was on top of everything. I was in control of everything around me. I couldn't remember that having happened to me ever before. In fact, I was always just the opposite. Very often, I was not in control of anything in my life. The chaos usually depressed me, and of course that depression drove me to food.

"Now, I hardly recognize myself. I take care of everything around me with plenty of time left over to go places and to do fun things. Even my car is clean and waxed all the time. I find it hard to believe."

Improvement in one area will effect improvement in other areas. Use your momentum to launch a real campaign to be in control of everything in your life.

Your environment helped you to get fat and to stay fat. Now that you are changing your patterns, search for anything that does not serve you well. Be honest in your search. Don't overlook anything. Just backing off a step or two will help you to make simple changes. Be the captain of your own ship. Be the master of what happens in your world. Replace stress situations with solutions that produce feelings of satisfaction. Take a little bit at a time, one step at a time. Give yourself the chance to grow.

Take your time. Don't be in a hurry. Keep an open mind so that you can think. Begin by examining your leisure-time activities. Then move on to your work and then to your relationships and to your fears. There is no better time than right now. Let the confidence that you have developed with your new eating behavior influence everything else. Master your environment slowly and methodically by having the courage to discard useless shelters.

SUBLIMINAL IMPRESSIONS

We can think of the mind as having two distinctly different functions. One is the function of reasoning that we use on command. It is the function of the reasoning mind to make choices and to guide us in a "reasoning" direction. It is that reasoning mind that is offended when we act contrary to its guidance. It is the reasoning mind that produces the guilt that warns us that something went wrong.

The other part of the mind function is the instinctual mind. The instinctual mind does not make decisions, nor does it respond to command. Rather, it is a kind of storage center for information gathered from the senses. You may think of it as a computer memory center. Information may be added to this memory center, but nothing may be taken away nor erased from the "tape" at will. However, information tends to fade with time, although it is all stored in the mind, perhaps unused for years and years. Forgotten memories.

Have you ever smelled an odor that immediately propelled your thoughts back to some place in your childhood? That was your instinctual memory identifying stored information. You may smell apple pie baking and find yourself reminiscing about a summer day at your grandmother's house. Or you may catch a quick glance of a canoe on top of a passing car and flash back to summer camp when you were eleven years old. Your instinctual memory is at work outside of your conscious control.

The instinctual memory records subliminal impressions. Those are impressions recorded on the mind without conscious awareness by some very sharp quick impression. That impression can then influence the reasoning mind when circumstances trigger that information. Fear of darkness or of dogs, of heights, or water, or of cigar-smoking men, or of anything, can be a reaction to information impressed subliminally on the instinctual memory. It is then sent back to the surface, into the reasoning, conscious mind, when circumstances provide the key to a particular coded shred of information. We cannot always control information available for storage.

Visual images make strong impressions on the instinctual memory, and much can be directly under your control. You can control what you choose to look at and what you choose to look away from. For instance, you may choose to pass over a dessert advertisement in a magazine, or look away from a food commercial on television, or avert your stare away from someone in a restaurant eating a baked potato covered with sour cream and butter. You are free to choose not to notice every ice cream shop that you pass during the day, or the pizza in the restaurant next to the dry cleaners. You may choose not to anticipate the assortment of candy in the lobby of the movies.

It is really not necessary to study the food section of the newspaper for food costs and recipes. If you collect food coupons, do it directly before you go out to shop (on a full stomach, of course). Try to get away from making those subliminal impressions on your mind. If you provide continuous food information for your instinctual memory, you will have too many food impressions ready to be uncoded whenever any situation reminds you of eating.

Don't dream of a day when you will be thin enough to eat as "normal" people eat. You are now eating as a normal person, and subliminal food impressions will keep you a prisoner of your false appetite forever. *Look away!* Think of other things. Subliminal impressions are very potent, so make every effort to monitor input. Make a habit of looking away and thinking of something else whenever you are confronted with food cues. It will become automatic with practice..

You are now in a kind of recovery stage. You have triumphed

in a battle and need to steady your nerves to gain strength. Like the recovering alcoholic who must keep alcohol out of the house and must avoid old haunts for a while, you must control situations that may have subliminal food impressions to tempt you to take "just one taste."

It is the mark of mature behavior to tune out all of the subliminal messages that you choose to tune out. Thin-thinking people have trained themselves to think of food only when they feel hungry. They control any impulse to eat until the proper time for a meal.

One of the staggering health problems in this country is the food-processing industry. Is it coincidence that Americans are overweight and undernourished? Our economy depends on the science of suggestion. You are being "programmed" to eat too much. If you want to be in control, you must "deprogram" your environment and choose to make choices with your reasoning mind.

Food commercials and advertisements on television and in magazines are masterfully deceptive. They speak to your subliminal mind, selling food as a secondary need. First, they sell happiness, group acceptance, sex, youth, and success. They appeal to your "desires." Then they address your appetite for food.

You may be sure that the food-processing industry, advertising its products, is not concerned about your health, nor the nutritional value of the product. Big business will package absolutely anything that you will buy. The next time you are in a market, read the ingredients listed on the package of a nationally advertised bakery treat. It seems really foolish to list the ingredients. They are all almost impossible to pronounce.

Monitor and control subliminal impression. You are the victim of a psychological, manipulative, deceitful movement to take your money and leave you holding an empty calorie. You are being fleeced with the old pickpocket's trick of focusing your attention on the left hand while the right hand quickly cleans out your pockets.

Advertisers know how to entice you to buy and to overeat, and they have all of the know-how to program your appetite. They have substituted psychological needs for your biological needs.

If you want to learn more about marketing and subliminal advertising, reserve one hour this week to go to a supermarket. Browse up and down the aisles reading labels and studying packages. Notice the effect of the displays. Don't buy anything, just study the marketplace. You will be fascinated with things that you have never noticed before. You will educate yourself. You will probably continue to research the power behind the "hidden persuaders."

Don't be victimized. Control information being fed to your instinctual memory. You are not going to avoid all insipid advertising, subliminal messaging, and fast-food garbage with snack stands on every corner, vending machines, and ubiquitous food-dispensing trucks. The food industry is a giant that is getting bigger every day to keep pace with a swelling population. Be aware of the influence, and to every underhanded, hidden message that you detect, add a little one of your own:

"I moved to Los Angeles from Boston last year to try my hand at acting. I figured that Los Angeles certainly was the place to either make it or break it in that field," reports William Jensen. "When I arrived in L.A., I couldn't believe the hot-dog stands, on almost every block. They were all shapes and all sizes, and each one had some kind of slogan that boasted of the uniqueness of the hot dog or the hamburger. I always loved a good hamburger. I was overwhelmed.

"My friends would occasionally speak of this or that 'famous' stand, and we would go there to sample the famous hamburgers. I tried hamburgers with chili oozing out between the buns and down my forearms. I tried hamburgers with peanuts, and with dates, and soy sauce and boysenberry jam, and, and, and—and you name it! All California burgers were made with lettuce, mayonnaise, and tomatoes and pickles anyway, so anything added was certain to totally eliminate the taste of meat. As a matter of fact, now that I think of it, none of these 'famous' stands was known for good meat, only the stuff that they put on it.

"Anyway, one day five months later and twenty pounds heavier, it dawned on me what was happening. Or, I should say, what I had let happen. At best, those famous stands served the closest thing to garbage that I had ever eaten, and they were famous because they served a big portion for a small price. I was wearing twenty pounds of the most inexpensive ingredients available—famous inexpensive ingredients.

"I was just able to focus it all one day. I was being fooled; no—I was fooling myself. I was caught up in the fun, and when I stopped to look back on it, it wasn't so much fun at that. Boy, I had no idea how strong outside suggestion to eat really was. When I realized it all, I began to pay attention to all the cues. It is unbelievable when you study it. Between the food and the eating advertising, the alcohol, the beer, and the wine advertisements, and the cigarette billboards, they, whoever 'they' may be, are telling us to get addicted. With television, magazines, newspapers, outdoor advertising, and signs of every variety, we hardly have a chance.

"It made me a little angry. Here I was fat and uncomfortable and I didn't know why, and I hadn't planned that it would happen.

"Well, I decided right then and there that I'd been had. I wasn't going to play the game any longer. I passed up all of those 'famous' hot-dog stands, and as I went by them, I thought of all the repulsive things that might be going on behind those counters. There was always something about every one of them that I had to purposely divert my attention from anyway, so it was easy for me to imagine unpleasant things. I could even imagine more unsanitary and unhealthy things about the stands that were not famous—after all, nobody was in charge there to keep an eye on things. You can imagine the fantasies I enjoyed. I even carried it over to television commercials and to other advertising. I became very expert at imagining unsanitary conditions wherever food was being handled and the detached people who were touching and retouching the food that I ate. I developed quite a case against the food establishment. I must admit that I may have carried it a bit too far at times. I arrived at the point where I wouldn't even buy canned foods. I couldn't stop my analysis, and all food processors became suspect. I've since relaxed a bit, but I don't eat anything without first reviewing how it got to me and what may have happened to it along the way.

"Now, whenever I notice a food place or a food ad, I am not attracted to it in the way that I used to be. I have reprogrammed myself. I feel much healthier and I enjoy being in control of my environment. Those slick food messages make me laugh a little disdainfully now."

Assert yourself! Understand the "enemy," so that you can prepare to conquer. You are exposed to food in more places than just in your kitchen and in the grocery market. Our environment is inundated with food. You are being influenced to overeat by way of your subconscious, that level of awareness just below the top. You are being baited to be hooked. The piper plays an enticing tune as he leads you into the land of no control.

AUTOSUGGESTION

It is very useful, again in a subliminal way, to go to sleep at night with a thought that is positive and is goal directed. We call this "autosuggestion" because it is suggestion directed to your subconscious mind by you yourself, just at the time that your conscious mind lets go to the subconsciousness of sleep.

Autosuggested thought is the last conscious thought at the end of a day of millions of different thoughts. It is that last bit of information planted in the mind that will be the first available information for recall.

Practice autosuggestion each night before you fall off to sleep. It will end your day on a positive note, and it will prepare you to sleep and to dream. There is no sense in wasting sleeping time. You can plant a thought each night before you slip into the hypnotic state of sleep, using that time to saturate the mind with soothing inspirational ideas and with positive reports of well-being.

The first thing to do to prepare for autosuggestion is to write exactly what it is you want to suggest. For instance, you might write that you want to suggest to your subconscious mind that you will stay in control, or that you will lose weight. Then, from that general idea, design a phrase that will communicate those thoughts directly and simply to your mind. The phrase or phrases must represent the entire thought, and must be simple enough to recall and to repeat every night in exactly the same

words. Write down many different treatments until you get the
one that is just right for you. Then write that phrase or sentence
over and over, perhaps twenty-five times, to test it and see if it
sounds effective with the repetition.

You might say, "I am in control of my own life, feeling thinner
every day and proud of myself." Or, "I am getting smaller with
my own control. I like myself and will always be kind to me." Or,
"I'm a success. I control my destiny. I will succeed in anything of
my choice."

Write as many different ways to say what you want to suggest
as you possibly can. Then review and select the single best one.
It should be clear, precise, and easy. When you have decided on
the sentence that best describes the feelings you want to incorporate into your subconscious mind, rehearse it during the day to
be sure that you can remember it. Repeat it exactly the same way
each time. Say it to yourself at every opportunity. Write it down
on some scrap paper or in the margin of your newspaper. Memorize it! Believe it!

The first night that you use your autosuggestion will set the
quality for all subsequent times. As with all new behavior, try to
lay the groundwork, the foundation, with care so that you may
build a sound structure. The returns are enormous.

Before you retire, take a shower. A bath is even better. Feel as
calm and as relaxed and serene as you can. Lie on your back in
bed with your head propped up comfortably and with your eyes
closed. Then inventory and relax all of your muscles from your
head—from the very top of your head—to the tips of your toes.
Start with the scalp and include every muscle of the face, neck,
shoulders, chest, back, belly, hips, arms, legs, every large and
small muscle of the body right down to and including the toes.
Tighten each muscle as you go, hold it tight for a moment, and
then release the tension. Move on to each and every muscle,
tensing and then releasing it. This simple relaxation exercise
will take no more than eight or ten minutes. After you relax each
muscle group—head, shoulders, arms, chest, abdomen, legs,
feet—take a slow, d-e-e-p breath. Hold that breath for a slow
count of ten and then exhale very s-l-o-w-l-y. Breathe deeply after tensing and relaxing each muscle group.

After you have relaxed your whole body and you feel comfortable and easy, whisper your autosuggestion sentence semiaudibly. Repeat the sentence slowly and precisely. After whispering the sentence five times, repeat it again without moving your lips and without voice. Repeat it to yourself, focusing the sound of your inner voice on an imaginary spot directly behind your closed eyes. Use your s-l-o-w, d-e-e-p breaths to time the repetition of your sentence. Listen to your breathing getting more steady with each breath, each time you fill your lungs with air. Listen and hear your sentence each time that you repeat it.

Repeat your magic sentence as many as fifty times, calmly and reassuringly, clearly focused behind your closed, relaxed eyes. You will be getting very sleepy. You will be fading to sleep with each s-l-o-w breath you breathe, and each time you hear your sentence telling you what you want to do. Say your sentence one last time, adjust your position, if you will, and drift off to sleep. You may find that you slip off to sleep long before you have completed your ritual.

This whole procedure, this life-giving ritual, takes very little time. Go through it every night. Approach it unhurriedly and concentrate on breathing, timing, and sentence repetition. Feel more relaxed and tired with each sentence and with each breath. Make a quick check every once in a while to be sure that all of your muscles remain free of tension. Release those that may have tightened. B-r-e-a-t-h-e s-l-o-w-l-y, exhale smoothly. Hear your words voiced with your inner voice behind your eyes in the dark, uncluttered spaces of your mind. Repeat your words the same way each and every time.

Make this autosuggestion a regular part of your life and you will develop a tremendous power of self-control. It is a life-giving ritual that may produce benefits far beyond your expectation. It may alleviate myriad psychosomatic suffering as a fringe benefit. You may change the suggestion when your needs change. For instance, you may have a job interview coming up. Your stature will be enhanced at the interview if you practice autosuggestion the night or two before. Design a phrase about why you should have the job, and about your confidence and superiority.

Autosuggestion is powerful. Use it as you would use an important tool. Treat it with respect and care to avoid diluting its power.

WALKING COMMITMENT

With the Mannix Method, any change from the usual that you have been asked to make has had a time limit and may terminate before you complete the twelve weeks of basic training.

The very strict rule of no protein for supper has been relaxed. The Food Journal has been eliminated. "Solo" eating has been adjusted. Now your commitment to walking each day is strictly a matter of your choice. The purpose in releasing you from the walking commitment is so that you may now function free of imposed rules and restrictions. Your new eating behavior has evolved and outgrown original foundation groundwork. You are now eating as an adult with self-control, without external regulation. In short, you are the master.

Be aware, however, that although the walking commitment is no longer required, it makes a great deal of sense to continue with some form of daily body movement. Walking is certainly one of the most pleasant.

Remember, too, that foods seem to be getting more caloric, and our modern world demands little physical movement. Caloric body fuel and no physical expenditure equals stored fat. You may either eat more simply with fewer gourmet delights, fleeting delights—or you may arrange to burn more calories. As in all things, the balance makes the difference.

Your food taste may have already changed appreciably to the lighter, healthier, fresher foods. If you continue to walk or perhaps start to exercise (see next session), you will achieve a good balance of body fuel and energy output to stay in optimum physical shape. Your psychological health is an extra!

It is your choice. Most people learn to really enjoy walking because it makes them feel wonderful. If you stop your walking, you will actually recognize a large difference in your feeling of well-being.

‌‌‌‌‌

‌‌‌

‌‌‌

‍‍

Food Management

Weight control is food management. It is now time to work out the details of a sound management plan. Most readers know that you cannot eat many starchy foods, or sugared foods, and maintain good health and a trim body. Common sense tells you that. You obviously cannot eat pasta all of the time and expect to maintain a sensible weight. That is especially true of individuals who gain weight very easily. So intelligent food management must dictate the right time for the right food. Once again, as in all things, balance and common sense define the territory.

Read the labels in the grocery store when you market. Don't buy food packaged with sugar. Why eat those hidden extra calories? For example, canned peas don't have to contain sugar. Yet most brands have sugar. Sugar is the surest way to rack up extra calories. And look out for sugar disguised as: dextrose, corn syrup, glucose, sucrose, and even honey.

Eliminating sugar is probably one of the wisest routes to good food management. If you hanker for sweet desserts, then you have all the more reason to eliminate the sugar in all of the other foods that you eat. You may then allow yourself a sensible portion of that extraspecial dessert in your favorite restaurant, or a piece of your mother's special lemon cake. You may feel free to enjoy it because you have eliminated the sugar unnecessarily added to other foods. You will have "banked" those nonessential calories equal to your special dessert. You will also minimize the risk of feeding a possible sugar addiction.

Read the labels on all packaged food. Buy the ones with the fewest empty calorie ingredients. You will find that sugar is the second major ingredient in most packaged food. It is also in many breads, some pasta, most canned vegetables, fruit drinks, and even baby food. It is difficult to understand why sugar is used so extensively in foods that aren't supposed to be sweet. Does the food industry anticipate larger and more continuous volume buying from sugar addicts? Let's hope not!

Refer to a calorie counter paperback book so that you may possibly avoid some unnecessary calories. If you have cookies in the house for the other family members, and you occasionally have a few after a meal, calculate your caloric investment. Buy those that have the fewest calories. Gingersnaps have less than half the calories of fig newtons. One brownie contains 243 calories, whereas a raised doughnut has 136 calories. Know and choose foods that allow you eating pleasure and at the same time represent calorie economy. Consume intelligently.

That approach to food is called management. It represents a knowledge of the various values of foods, much the way you know the value of the different coins that make up the dollar. Then exercise mature healthy eating habits, and manage sensible food selection. That is the formula for controlling your weight. It takes some close attention to lose extra pounds, but once you are the way you want to be, it is easy and very rewarding to stay in the driver's seat.

FASTING

Don't make the mistake of fasting to lose weight. The weight that appears to vanish is only water, and it will return promptly when you resume eating.

Fasting for even one day can be extremely harmful, especially if you don't drink sufficient liquid. You may choose not to nourish your body, but your need for vitamins, minerals, and protein is ever present. Once the body has exhausted the stored supply of blood sugar, it turns to the most easily converted body tissue for food. In a sense, you consume yourself to supply the brain with nutrients and the body with sufficient energy. The very first body tissue that is tapped is lean muscle. The lean muscles are the easiest to convert into blood sugar. Your heart is your leanest muscle. That should rest the case against indiscriminate fasting. Will you run even a remote risk of damaging your heart?

The liver can store a twenty-four-hour supply of blood sugar before your system uses itself for nourishment. You may therefore presume that a one-day fast will not be too risky for your health. It will not, however, assist in weight loss. It may actually result in just the opposite effect, after water has been replenished and your appetite satisfied.

If you want to fast for one day to rest your body from the continuous processing of food, and maybe to practice discipline, do it properly. First, get an okay from your doctor. He may want to examine you before he gives his permission. Follow his instructions. Fasting for even one day may be risky for some people, and only your doctor knows for sure. And please remember that the night before a fast should not be a Roman orgy. A small supper of cooked vegetables is best, and a restful night of sleep is important.

Begin your fasting day with a large glass of water. Then be sure to drink ten or twelve glasses of water during the day. It is my opinion that one should drink fruit juice during any fast. That will not violate the fast, but will be supplying a source of blood sugar periodically to relieve body stress. It may be good to fast one day every two weeks, with oranges three times during the day and with plenty of water and diluted fruit juices. It feels very good to empty fat cells for the day. It seems to create a nice buoyant feeling. The days following a fast require a very careful choice of food; stick close to light fruits, vegetables, and dairy products.

Anticipate and plan for a fast day. If Thursday is a fast day for you, as you approach Thursday, you will become psychologically prepared for a day without eating. Once you begin the fast, see it through until the following morning. The feeling of accomplishment that next morning will be worth the possible few moments of self-pity during abstinence.

Fasting is a test in self-discipline. It can be trying at first. Think about it before you try it. It is no great loss if you don't try it at all, but it is beneath you to try and not see it through. The mind has clever ways of compromising when you think you are deprived, as you well know. So approach fasting aggressively, with no room for excuses and lapses of memory. If you have decided not to eat during the day, a handful of peanuts or half a sandwich during the afternoon or in the evening is taboo. Fasting means not eating solid food all day. Don't try it unless you are prepared to make it through.

One of my clients, Max Vincent, relates his first fasting experience: "It wasn't until I'd finished the Mannix Method that I felt confident enough to try a day of fasting. In the past, whenever I heard one of my skinny health-food friends talking about fasting for a day, I used to be quite envious of that self-control and discipline. So I would eat something extra just to eradicate the idea. Anyway, after I was happy with the control that I had gained over my eating and had lost enough weight to feel good about myself, I thought it was time to try not eating for a day.

"It was difficult for me to consider what I was doing that first time. It was all I could do to comprehend that I wouldn't be eating for twenty-four hours. I had no lofty purpose for cleansing my body. I was really a little scared, if the truth be known.

"The night before, I had some steamed cauliflower with melted cheese sauce, some chicken broth, and herb tea. I had the feeling that I was in some kind of training. It seemed like a good idea to have a little protein so that I wouldn't be my usual hungry in the morning. The hot soup and the tea were to help me with a good night's sleep.

"I woke up like an electric light bulb in the morning. My eyes opened wide and didn't shut again. I was instantly awake. The first thing that I did was to take a cold shower. I have never taken a cold shower in my life before. I couldn't believe it. I just wanted to take my mind off the possibility of feeling hungry. Boy, I was acting crazy. Now that I look back on it, it was a real comedy scene, but at the time, I felt fear.

"After my painful experience in the water, I made a cup of herb tea. I was advised not to have any caffeine, and I sat down to read the morning paper before I left for work. I'm pretty lucky. I live alone and there was no one using food around me to tempt me to eat. I felt really confident then. I wasn't the least bit tempted to have anything to eat, and I didn't feel hungry, the way I usually do in the morning. It made me feel very disciplined and happy with myself. I was looking forward to the rest of the day when I left for work.

"I had a busy morning and I didn't think about eating once. At lunchtime, I had planned a tennis game with one of the guys in the office, and afterward I had a large glass of diluted grapefruit juice. I still wasn't feeling hungry enough to eat. I couldn't believe it! It was the longest time that I'd been without food in all of my life. I was in the driver's seat!

"I had a little trouble at dinnertime but I talked it over with myself. I was determined not to eat, and I knew that the only reason I was feeling hungry just then was because it was the regular time to eat. I had worked with all that during my training. It was an external cue to eat and I wasn't going to buy it! I took a hot bath and went out to a play at a small theater in my neighborhood.

"When I came home and was preparing for bed, I knew that I had made it. I was so proud of myself. I felt terrific, almost high. I went through my relaxation ritual and I fell off to sleep quickly.

"The next morning was another big surprise. I thought that I would be ravenous for breakfast, but instead I couldn't really decide whether I was hungry at all. I waited until after my shower and I dressed before I went into the kitchen to get breakfast. I was beginning to feel a little hunger, so I prepared some fresh fruit and some yogurt and I ate very leisurely. I just didn't want any more. I felt terrific.

"The experience was so wonderful for me that I am now fasting one day every week. I always do it on the same day, of course, and each time I experience the same marvelous feeling."

I hear many similar stories. A one-day fast can be a delightful experience if you prepare yourself for it and you don't do it to lose weight. It is a physical and mental cleansing that can do nice things for you. Some authorities recommend breaking fast with some form of roughage like salad or miller's bran. Try a salad for breakfast the morning following a fast, with some fresh broiled fish. If you want to give fasting a try, groom yourself for it and do your utmost for your best. Or perhaps fasting is not for you. Make your decision "to do" or "not to do" without anxiety. Always keep in mind that anxiety, with its attendant guilt and punishment, is a shelter of your childish past and will never again be a part of your mature existence. You've come a long way from being your own hangman.

SUMMARY

Throughout the Mannix Method, you have been working on the skills to eliminate destructive and negative addiction. It started with recognition, then with understanding. *Know thyself* is basic in your Mannix training. You were then directed to concentrate on an appreciation of life's many wonders.

You were guided to changes in attitude and in your environment so that childish shelters could be replaced. It is wise to be prepared to substitute healthy pleasures for discarded addiction. It is not enough to just give an addiction up. It might not have been a source of great pleasure, but it was a source of feeling, albeit destructive. Without those feelings that come with addiction, you may think you feel alone and devoid of pleasure. It is necessary, therefore, to find alternate sources of fulfillment, positive sources of pleasure that permit you to evolve toward peace of mind and a feeling of completeness. Be on guard against boredom and inertia.

Finding positive, rewarding addictions will be worth every bit of your effort so that you may experience "real" satisfaction. You must find things that don't produce self-condemnation, that old familiar emotional whipping devil. You must look for things that you may experience every day for a continuous supply of pleasure and satisfaction.

Games, in general, are poor sources of tranquil pleasure. Most of them require a competitive appetite with the winner-and-loser theme. Perhaps the chance of you being the loser is just enough to diminish your pleasure.

At the start, find some activity that you do by yourself. Find something you don't have to be good or bad at, to win or to lose. Find something that is privately yours with personal benefits. Take an ideal opportunity to develop a new rewarding addiction with walking. You may try to run now that you have decreased your body load and have increased your strength. Swimming, yoga, meditation, story writing, sewing, knitting, needlepoint, or playing musical instruments are all naturals. Find sources of private pleasure to replace the all-too-brief and unhealthy rewards of overeating.

HIGHLIGHTS

A. Boredom

1. Boredom breeds obsession. Obsessive thoughts beget compulsive actions like binge eating.
2. Activity overpowers food thinking.
3. Activity and productivity give real emotional satisfaction.

Commit yourself by signing the following contract.

Remember that this is a point of honor—a private obligation to yourself:

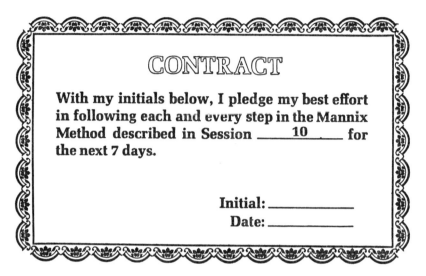

CONTRACT

With my initials below, I pledge my best effort in following each and every step in the Mannix Method described in Session ____10____ for the next 7 days.

Initial: _____
Date: _____

4. Boredom may be built into your daily routine.
5. Frustration, anger, disappointment, depression, and eating thoughtlessly are all the offspring of boredom.

B. Control and Deception

1. Control in one area will have a domino effect on all areas of your life.
2. Control gathers momentum extending to every part of your life.
3. Control is undermined with self-deception.
4. Self-deception is dishonest.
5. Self-deception puts you out of control.
6. Self-deception is a childish shelter.

C. Brain Functioning

1. The brain functions with the reasoning mind and the instinctual memory.

2. The reasoning mind selects, guides, judges, controls.
3. The instinctual mind stores information in automatic fashion.
4. Subliminal impressions may send information without the awareness of the reasoning mind.
5. Visual recognition strongly impresses the instinctual memory.
6. Food advertising uses subliminal suggestion.

D. *Autosuggestion*

1. Autosuggestion is positive, goal-directed thought before sleep.
2. Autosuggestion works best with ritual repetition of simple, clear messages.
3. Autosuggestion works best combined with breathing and relaxation techniques.
4. Autosuggestion gets better with daily practice. It is powerful, to be treated with respect.

E. *Walking Commitment*

1. Conclude your commitment to walk, if you wish.
2. Consider walking as a permanent part of your healthy life.
3. Understand that walking provides enjoyment while balancing body function.

F. *Food Management*

1. Understand food management to control weight.
2. Make a sound management plan. Know your foods. Know your limits.
3. Eliminate unnecessary hidden calories.
4. Strive to provide healthy body fuel.

G. *Fasting*

1. Fasting does not produce weight loss.
2. Fasting can be dangerous. Consult your doctor.

3. Fasting forces the body to consume muscle tissue such as the heart.
4. Fasting can be pleasant for one day with proper management.
5. Fasting must include liquid and possibly fruit in lieu of nothing.
6. Fasting exercises self-discipline.

H. Weight Chart

1. Record and graph your weight.
2. Allow your weight to be lost gradually, naturally.

I. Time for Session 10

One week, as usual.

SESSION 11

Finish Strong

This session is the last seven-day training session. You have realized some of your enormous potential and know now that you are a rich reservoir of virtually untapped talent. You can do almost anything you want to, if you commit yourself to the task. You can take one giant step and then another and another—and the secret is that you take them one at a time, believing in yourself.

Finish this week with meticulous care. Practice Tapered Eating without deviation for the next seven days. Perhaps at this point in training time, you have amended Tapered Eating here and there to suit your own personal life-style. Return now, for this eleventh week, to following Tapered Eating exactly. You may have forgotten how vibrant and healthy it makes you feel.

Like autosuggestion, this final information saturating your instinctual memory will always be the most easily recalled. Begin a review of the Mannix Method with a serious sense of purpose and of accomplishment. Live today, tomorrow, and every day of this week, training yourself with a kind of inspired application. Guarantee that the last layer of modified behavior serves your best interest with an abundance of positive reinforcement and energy. Be totally and always aware of your long-term values. Guard against lethargy or diluted motivation. Make this week's practice nothing short of perfection, so that your Mannix behavior becomes naturally automatic. Give anything extra you can muster now, so that you finish strong. Remember, a racer who finishes strong doesn't do anything *different* to end the race; she/he just concentrates a little harder on stride and style to do just what she/he has been doing all along. She/he does what she/he has been doing *better*. Athletes know that strong finishers are winners.

THE TEN-PERCENT INVESTMENT

Everything that you eat and everything positive that you do for your body is an investment. Your life, in the main, is a product of what you want to make it, what your mind is willing to make of it. The quality of your living will depend almost totally on your perception of how it can be. How much are you willing to spend to maintain your investment?

If you spend a mere ten percent of your time maintaining your investment, you will improve the other ninety percent of your time to its peak efficiency. Just ten percent, less than two and a half hours a day, to improve the other twenty-one and a half hours. A very small expenditure to secure the greatest return on the most important investment of your life. Simply consider the maintenance of your person one of life's necessities.

Two and a half hours a day set aside for taking care of your being are all that you need to keep you in the pink. Most people are willing enough to give every waking hour to repairing the damaged self, should illness befall. It is simple wisdom that an ounce of prevention is worth a pound of cure. Not only is the ten-percent investment wise, it is enjoyable.

Thirty minutes to eat each of your meals adds up to one and a half hours a day. That's a basic requirement for good health, good nutrition, good control, and good body and mind maintenance. Don't leave the table before thirty minutes have passed unless you are leaving food on your plate. Table rules are that you put your fork down after each bite, that you chew slowly and swallow your food completely before you lift the fork again. Relax when you eat. Use fork replacement and slow chewing to help you eliminate any sense of time emergency that you happen to bring to the table. Exercise *control!* Pace yourself! If you feel like rushing or like shoveling a few forkfuls into your mouth quickly, *control* the impulse. Purposely exaggerate the slow-down until any excitement settles. Remember, *timing* affects *outcome.* That's true about many things in your life. Don't think of the thirty-minute rule as imposed regulation. You are fully aware of its great contribution to maintaining control. Consider it part of the ten-percent investment. Know it as something that you do every time you sit down to eat. Understanding nurtures acceptance. This one ounce of behavior will save you many pounds of cure!

Take *two intermissions* whenever you eat anything, and always *leave at least two bites* of food on the plate. Observe these two rules without fail. They take no planning and little effort. In the frenzy of emotional binging, should that ever happen again, exercise those simple techniques even though they don't seem to make a bit of difference at the time. They will summon your control center to keep you on guard. They really will make every difference. Make them habit for life. They are a part of your ten-percent investment!

Another easy and effective technique to insist on at all times is to *delay starting* to eat for one minute when a plate is put before you. Take a deep breath and relax yourself for sixty short seconds before you taste the food. Merely good table manners. Allow yourself to get used to the *idea* of eating for a minute, before you start to eat. It somehow gives you the time to organize your other eating techniques. Once you have permanently incorporated the "one-minute delay" rule into all of your food encounters, you will always be reminded that eating involves control to be healthy and enjoyable.

Don't ever talk with your fork in your hand. Good table manners will help you to think about what and how fast you are eating. So simple! Of course, you are fully aware now of the fact that the most important techniques for staying healthy and thin are everyday common-sense procedures.

One word of caution. *Wait for a full thirty minutes after any meal* if you entertain the thought of eating something that isn't scheduled for you. You may finish dinner at someone's home and find yourself anticipating some delicious homemade cake. Give yourself thirty minutes before you permit yourself a piece of that cake. After those thirty minutes, discuss with yourself the need for the cake once again. Usually you will find that your desire has vanished and your healthy feeling of control has superseded. If, however, you still want a piece of cake after thirty minutes, you will be able to eat it with control and with no risk of reaching for a second piece with the ensuing guilt.

Try to recall the table manners and eating etiquette that were part of your young life. Everyone at the dining table usually waited until everyone was served before beginning to eat (the one-minute delay). Many families often had a moment's silence before eating, which again delayed beginning to eat. No one talked with a full mouth, nor with eating utensils in hand. Arms were relaxed near your body to pace eating. No one left the table until everyone was finished (pacing), and dessert and coffee were served well after a meal was finished and very often in another room. The eating procedure was slow and relaxed. You see, you are not restricting yourself in any way, you are returning to a more elaborate style of eating. You are returning to one of the basics of days gone by.

Become a gourmet. Eat deliberately, savoring the taste of each bite of food. Never mix the tastes of different foods in the same bite. Wait until you have finished with the sensation of one taste before you take another mouthful. Eating is an experience that can thrill the senses and delight the imagination. Enjoy the experience. Stuffing food into your mouth the way hamburgers, sandwiches, and cookies are devoured is certainly not truly enjoying the food that you think that you like best. If you don't like to eat, stuffing food into your mouth rapidly is, of course, as good a way as any to obtain nutrients. But people who don't like to eat don't abuse food, as a rule, nor do they appreciate it, nor do they overeat—nor do they get fat.

Make your food last as long as you can, and check yourself frequently to feel if you have had enough. Always finish eating a meal feeling a little less than stuffed rather than feeling uncomfortable with "one more bite for the road." The worst thing that can happen is that you may feel slightly hungry a little sooner than you expect later on. Stop eating one bite before you are full to feel your appestat and to avoid going on to a binge. If you eat beyond your stop signal, you will supply more blood sugar than your system needs, which in turn will call for more insulin to prevent sugar richness in your blood. Extra insulin will make you feel hungry or unsatisfied although you are physically full. If you stop eating at the first sign of satiety, you will not lose control, and as a result of being in control, you will not feel inflated nor will you become fat.

You know all of the techniques. You have acquired and practiced the skills necessary for losing weight and keeping you thin. You have proved that the Mannix Method works. The "know-how" is your property. Only ten percent of your time is now necessary to maintain your self-respect and the healthy body in which that respect is housed. What a small price to pay for the liberation from childish shelters.

EXERCISE

If you do some kind of exercise for one hour each day to complete the time allotted to your ten-percent maintenance of your investment, you will never again have to worry about your weight!

What is exercise? Exercise is defined by Webster as habitual activity. It does not have to be strenuous, exhausting, punishing, or distasteful to be beneficial. But it must be habitual to improve body function and to regulate metabolism. And it must be enjoyable to become a good habit.

Exercise should not be considered a way to lose weight. One hour of any exercise will not burn up sufficient calories to offset a small piece of chocolate cake after dinner. However, exercise is a superb way to equalize the differences in your daily food consumption, so that you may have that occasional piece of chocolate cake without having to worry about growing the "bulge and tire" from it. More important than balancing your energy supply/demand, exercise will make you feel physically healthy and mentally disciplined. You won't have any difficulty controlling weight as long as you continue your newly learned eating behavior patterns.

Continue walking. It is an ideal exercise for everybody. Walking uses almost all of the muscles in the body and is especially important for the cardiovascular system. The movement in walking accelerates breathing and improves blood circulation. More oxygen is supplied to all cells, and wastes, impurities, and fats are forced out of their comfortable attachment to tissue. As you have probably discovered, a short walk will allay feelings of hunger. The digestive process stops, the pulse quickens. The stress of walking is beneficial. Walking revitalizes. It also increases the oxygen supply to the brain, making it function more efficiently. All organs function better with a larger supply of oxygen.

So *walking*, like all exercise, will make you feel better physically and mentally. If you establish the attitude that it is part of your maintenance investment, and you make time to walk each and every day, it will surely become one of your favorite habits. In a sense, you will become addicted to something healthy for the mind and the body.

If you walk briskly and you cover a mile or more, after a while you may want to consider running. Don't begin running without having your doctor check you out thoroughly. Even if you feel better than you have ever felt in your life, get a checkup and tell your doctor that you are planning to start running. Ask for his okay. You may feel and look terrific and still benefit from a checkup. This is a must; see your doctor.

If you want to run, you must have the proper frame of mind. If you are thrilled with walking and look to running to further enjoyment and to heighten your experience, you are thinking in the right direction. Running is something a little short of meditation and it can be definitely addictive. Running does wonderful things for both your physical and your mental well-being. You must run every other day for perhaps a month, then run every day for six to eight months or even a year, before you fall in love with it. It is a long-term investment with untold rewards, if you aren't impatient.

Running fits in well with the training methods that you used to control your weight. Becoming a runner is a training process, starting with the one-day-at-a-time approach until it becomes automatic and you develop a need to run. When that happens, you will never have to budget your time to run again. More than likely, you will have to tear yourself away from running to work or to eat, or to do household chores. Running becomes an addiction. The time that you spend running will be private time for you only. You can't run and remain anxious or frustrated. So running time is pure therapy. It is time away from daily trials and tribulations.

Runners say that the peace of mind they enjoy while they run is maintained for hours afterward. That explains why runners prefer to finish the day with a run. Those people claim that it revitalizes them after a long day and calms them down to enjoy the evening and sleep.

Runners report less use of alcohol, sugar, tobacco, starch, drugs, and heavy food after they develop an addiction to running. It is not uncommon for a runner to have a heartbeat half that of a normal rate, and to need less sleep to achieve the same rest. They all attest to improved concentration and memory.

Addicted runners have an abundance of self-confidence. They seem sure of themselves because they demonstrate self-discipline, control, and purpose.

If you want to give running a try, the first thing to do is to buy a pair of shoes designed specifically for running. They are available in many shoe stores, sporting-goods stores, department stores, and some general stores. They range in price from ten to fifty dollars. Buy the best that you can afford. Proper shoes will make the difference between running and bouncing up and down. A good comfortable "professional" shoe will contribute to your joy in running.

Before you buy your shoes, decide on the running place. The surface that you will run on will determine the shoe style for you. After you have picked out the kind of surface that you will be running on, consult your shoe salesperson for a recommendation. The salesperson is an expert, and will show you shoes designed specifically for your terrain, your experience, and your budget.

You can run almost anywhere. The softer surfaces (like grass) are easier on your feet and legs. If you must run on pavement, try to find streets that are smooth. Minimize distractions so that you can concentrate on running. Select minimal traffic times to avoid exhaust fumes. Runners share a kind of unspoken respect and fraternity. They will quickly accept you. And don't be concerned with the passersby in cars. Running is only for you. You don't have to please anybody. It is totally noncompetitive. Professional racers don't compete against anyone else. They run against their own records, they challenge their own endurance to extend their training. They aren't out to be better than anyone but themselves. They want to grow better. Does that fit your train of thought?

Find loose, lightweight clothing. Make sure that the legs of your pants or shorts are loose around the thighs. Wear a T-shirt without sleeves, so that you are not too warm. It may feel chilly before you begin running, but five minutes later you will be warm and sweating. You will be comfortable running in temperatures down to freezing if there is no wind, but brisk wind can drive the chill factor down drastically.

Run alone until you establish some distance and then run with occasional company. You will become more easily addicted if you run alone.

A good way to begin running, after you have prepared yourself, is to measure off one mile. Use the odometer in your car, or consult veteran runners, or carry one of those inexpensive counters that hang from your waist. Begin by walking briskly for the first quarter of the mile, then running the next quarter, and walking the next and running the last. Use the walk-run method for two weeks.

Next, divide the mile up into thirds. For two weeks run, walk, and run in thirds. You must push yourself to make running progress. After one month of the run-walk routine, try only running without walking. Start running only a half mile for two or three weeks, or until you are running easily and you think that it is time to increase distance. Then run one mile. Get ready to increase your running to one mile by marking a date on your calendar a week or more in advance. The night before the one-mile run, have a very light supper and go to bed early. Run the whole mile. Push yourself to make progress. You are sufficiently trained to run the mile. The exuberance that you feel at the finish will put you on the way to being a runner. Beyond this one-mile point, you will know what to do by yourself. You will know another victory.

A few hints may be in order: Don't run on the balls of your feet; the heels hit first. Develop your stride for long, steady leg movements. It is beneficial to spend time during each run concentrating exclusively on your body movement.

Use your arms, with your hands above the elbows, to help pull your legs forward and to take some of the weight off your knees. As you run, you will see how the arms move naturally in time with the legs. As you concentrate on your body movement, coordinate arm movement carefully into your stride to help move you along.

Check, every once in a while, to be sure that you are relaxed while running. Especially check shoulders and buttocks, because they are usually the first areas to tighten. Running will be more difficult if you aren't relaxed.

Breathe through both your nose and your mouth. Be aware of your breathing. Take deep, even breaths. Blow a little more air out than you take in. The muscles under stress produce a waste called lactic acid that is expelled through the lungs. Exhale forcibly to clear the lungs of this waste matter and to help keep the muscles limber and healthy. You may notice a sour taste or odor in your mouth after running. That's lactic acid. Brush your teeth or use a mouthwash after your run, because the odor tends to remain for some time.

Breathing properly is extremely important for running successfully. Learn to time breathing with your body movement. Some runners like to take two short breaths in and one forced breath out. They say that it meshes in well with their stride. In whatever way that you are comfortable breathing, work on a nice, easy, deep cadence.

One last point: As you run, your heart and breathing will accelerate in response to your body's increased demand for oxygen. Your oxygen supply system (heart and lungs) will go through stages to meet increasing demand for oxygen. During the first stage supply will be considerably less than demand, and the first part of the run will therefore be difficult. You may get out of breath and feel heavy and tired. Run through this period, to experience what runners call a "second wind." That "second wind" will be the gap closing between the body's demand for more oxygen and the supply system meeting the demand more efficiently. In a mile run, you may only have to go through one stage, or one second wind. As you increase running time to cover more distance, you may go through two or three stages of altering oxygen demand and supply. Perfect balance is usually reached after thirty minutes of running, and that's when addiction starts. That is when your mind as well as your muscles are flooded with oxygen and you experience a kind of euphoria. If you have the discipline to train, running will keep you healthy and "high," and thin for the rest of your life. You will be addicted for life, to life.

Swimming is said to be the best of all exercise. It is certainly the best for obese people because adipose tissue (fat) floats. Obese people can feel they are half their weight when in water.

If you are still too heavy for "exercising," and you would like a change of pace from your daily walk, try swimming. Any local church-sponsored community center usually has a pool that is open to the community at reasonable cost. At open-swim times there is an instructor on duty to help you to plan a training program.

Swimming shares many of the same principles as running. It is more precise, however, and much more graceful. Breathing and movement are still the most important components, and oxygen supply and demand are restraining forces. Again, approach a swimming regimen slowly. Swim two or three laps, then rest. Kick at the side of the pool until your legs are tired, then rest again. Swim another two laps and quit for that day. Add one lap at a time at your own pace. Work on breathing, because once you master that, you will be able to add laps with surprising rapidity.

Swimming shapes beautiful trim figures. You must be comfortable in the water, and have access to a pool, to develop addiction to swimming. It is a marvelous refreshing exercise that produces the same kind of euphoric reaction that running does when oxygen flows abundantly through the body system.

* * *

Bicycling can be a good form of exercise if you pedal more than you coast. When you are coasting, you are resting. A stationary bicycle in a gym provides almost as rigorous a workout as running. If you work at bicycling, it is a fine form of exercise and can be combined with travel and exploring interesting places that are a bit farther away than your walk has taken you.

Tennis is primarily a competitive game that provides exercise. It tones the muscles and improves your cardiovascular efficiency, but you must guard against the demeaning of self. If you are able to find partners, which is another of the problems with tennis, and can enjoy the exercise despite performance that falls short of perfection, it may well be the thing that delights you.

Golf is a good form of exercise if you stay out of a golf cart. What so often happens, however, is that people take to golf to be out walking in the fresh air. As soon as the game "bites" them, they spend most of their time criticizing themselves, trying to force relaxation, and riding the cart to get to the next shot faster. You can develop golf as a pleasant, addictive form of conditioning if you don't fall prey to feelings of frustration and discouragement.

Stretching, bending, twisting in a gymnasium is a terrific way to keep your muscles toned, but it isn't much fun.

However, if you persevere with floor exercises, and learn to isolate and develop separate muscles and muscle groups, you have a pleasurable feeling of accomplishment. It is an ideal way to condition your figure, but must be brisk and demanding to affect the cardiovascular system.

Of course you can exercise at home, but it is more easily done with other people. Set a time specifically to do exercises each day. If you are casual and plan to exercise when time becomes available, that time seldom comes. Set up a schedule or join an exercise class. Or form a small group of your own to meet every day at the same time and even the same place.

Weight lifting is generally for young men with no excess flesh. As a matter of fact, lifting weights is recommended for men who are too thin. It builds heavy muscle. If you are overweight, you don't want to translate rather buoyant fat into solid muscle. It will certainly make weight loss more difficult, and at a certain point almost impossible.

It is in vogue now for women to exercise with weights. Fortunately, hormones prevent women from developing heavy muscle. Use light weights and lift them many times. In doing any exercise, use weights light enough to be able to repeat the movement fifteen times.

As with any exercise, the going is slow at first. Plan lifting weights every other day for at least six months before you notice any improvement. Once you tone your muscles with weights, it is relatively easy to maintain muscle tone.

Weight lifting should not be done every day. The way that it affects muscle is interesting: You do not develop muscle when you lift against weight. In a sense, you injure the muscle and tear it down. Development is in the process of repair. The muscles repair themselves when they are rested, and become stronger to withstand the next assault. It is wise to skip a day in between weight-exercise days.

Weight exercisers usually pursue another form of exercise on days off from weights. Running or swimming is ideal for those in-between days. Working with weights tends to tighten and to stiffen muscles. Running and swimming loosen and stretch muscles. The combination is effective. Always consult your gym attendant to plan the right program for you; she or he is an expert and takes pride in advising you properly.

Many individual ball games are excellent ways to exercise; handball, racquet ball, squash. These are the high-energy-output games that burn many calories. Businessmen who sit all day and must entertain frequently turn to this quick, demanding exercise form.

Racquet-ball courts have been springing up everywhere in the last few years, and you can rent a paddle and court inexpensively. Try it. You can play from the very first time that you set foot on a court, and it's really fun!

* * *

It is possible to maintain reasonable weight with no exercise. It is certainly more difficult, but can be done. If you are incapacitated, food management and healthy behavior will suffice. Barring unusual circumstances, however, the opportunity to enjoy the extraordinary feelings that exercise provides should not be denied.

Habits are very comforting. You have proven that. Even overeating was dependent on the feeling of security that familiar procedures provide. So you know you are a natural for developing routine. Your new eating patterns again reinforce routine behavior. So seize the chance to become addicted to your own special flavor of exercise. There is variety enough to satisfy any preference.

Maintain your investment! One and a half hours a day are spent on fueling your body, and one hour each day must be devoted to using your body. You will be in control of a life that affords incredible enjoyment.

Be patient looking for the rewards from an exercise program. With any form of exercise, it takes time to develop proficiency, and then it takes some more time to develop positive dependency. The goal is to get the exercise habit, to be positively addicted to the positive, so that you may replace destructive addiction. Exercise can become habit if you choose something that is noncompetitive and you plan to give it one hour each day. Concentrate on movement and make it pleasant. Pleasure addicts. Start slow and easy and give yourself time to "hang into it."

You may not fall in love with exercise immediately if the whole idea is new. Trust that the effect, given a few months, will convert you totally.

Forced unpleasant exercise may help to balance calories, but the psychological damage done inventing clever avoidance techniques may set you back, to your detriment. You can never again afford to practice deceptive, childish behavior patterns that may infect the healthy parts of your life.

Remember that addiction takes time to develop. Positive addiction takes an even longer time to root than the negative kind, because it is goal oriented and very often not immediately gratifying. Negative addiction usually offers escape from reality, while the rewards gained from positive addiction require a mature understanding of yourself and your world.

Until you decide on a particular form of exercise, stay with walking. Don't begin to "exercise" until you really want to and are able to look forward to the daily performance with pleasure.

Take one hour a day to maintain your physical being as an investment in your healthy future and your vital now. If you plan to postpone exercise, use that hour for some other thing that can help the physical you. Consider yoga, massage, relaxation techniques, Jacuzzi, steam baths—anything that keeps you in touch with your physical dwelling place. Groom your mind for exercise later on if not right now. When you are ready to extend your physical hour to something more demanding, take on as much as makes you comfortable. Don't run the mile, or swim ten laps, or take an hour class. Do less than you think you are capable of at first, and then progress at your own pace, trusting yourself.

The ten-percent investment! Invest a mere ten percent of your

Commit yourself by signing the following contract.

Remember that this is a point of honor—a private obligation to yourself:

CONTRACT

With my initials below, I pledge my best effort in following each and every step in the Mannix Method described in Session ____11____ for the next 7 days.

Initial: _____

Date: _____

time for mind and body maintenance and you will be investing in your health, your beauty, and your psychological balance. So little to give for so much. Most of us use more time than that to run unnecessary errands.

SUMMARY

You are now on the last stretch to the finish line. Take pride in your achievement. You have changed the quality of your total life with a bag full of well developed living skills. Those skills assist you to delay momentary gratification for mature satisfaction. Those skills assist you to change that which can be changed to build a solid foundation of self-worth and self-respect.

HIGHLIGHTS

A. Finish Strong

  1. Winners finish strong.

B. The Ten-Percent Investment

   1. Invest two and a half hours a day to make the other twenty-one and a half hours better.
   2. Invest one and a half hours to fuel the body.
   3. Invest one hour to move the body.

C. Consider Exercise

   1. Exercise is habitual activity.
   2. Exercise need not be strenuous.
   3. Exercise can become a daily habit.
   4. Exercise should be noncritical, noncompetitive.
   5. Exercise to stay healthy, not to lose weight.
   6. Walking is one of the best forms of exercise.
   7. Running may evolve from walking.
   8. Swimming has many devotees.
   9. Bicycling may be deceptive.
  10. Tennis may break the spirit.

11. Golf is good if you walk and stay relaxed.
12. Floor exercises tone muscle.
13. Weight lifting is for the fit and thin.
14. Racquet ball, handball, squash, burn calories.
15. Make progress patiently. Concentrate on movement.
16. Become addicted. Stay with it for rewards.
17. Exercise to live better and to maintain your best investment.

D. Weight Chart

Weigh yourself and graph weight on chart.

E. Time for Session 11

One week for Session 11, as usual.

SESSION 12

Bon Voyage

You have completed the Mannix Method. Use your new behavior whenever you are involved with food. Remember, the last impression made on your instinctual memory is the first information to be recalled to influence behavior. Make your skills automatically available by using them constantly.

Adhere to Tapered Eating as a basic rule of behavior. Amend the style whenever you choose, but recognize that the deviation is the exception to the rule and should happen infrequently. If you find that you have deviated from this rule too many times, *do not diet* to get rid of those extra few pounds, anticipating that you will return to a sensible schedule as soon as you compensate for the extra weight. If you deviate from Tapered Eating a few too many times and it shows up on the scale, *calmly* and with deliberation go back to the tapering style, and follow it meticulously. Above all, *don't panic* when you gain a few pounds as the result of a round of closely spaced dinner parties, or family holidays, or just unusual circumstances. Resist the temptation to fast for one day to shed those few unwanted pounds. Don't allow feelings of guilt to send you into the panic of making "weight" decisions instead of "wait" decisions. Waiting means patience and control. Our Puritan grooming may motivate us to goals that are unrealistically rigid. The condition built on this attitude is called cognitive claustrophobia. Training is a process, not a happening. Deal with each day as a part of the whole structure of your life. Avoid self-deprecation with its inevitable failure behavior.

Resist extra trips to the scale on days when you feel stuffed. If you feel fat and you can trace that feeling to a recent occasion when you altered Tapered Eating, you don't need the scale to validate the feeling. That will only become a punitive action, and why volunteer for depression?

The scale should be a guide to help direct your eating plans for the day. That is all the scale is—it is a guide. It is not a monitor for reward, nor for punishment. The scale just indicates what you already know. If you eat a pizza dinner late one night, do not expect the scale to say you're sorry and home free the next morning. You know that you ate, so stay away from the scale if you think you have gained a few pounds. Stay off the scale until you feel closer to your best.

Weigh yourself only once a week until you have achieved your desired weight. Once you have realized your goals, use the scale each day, if you wish. Permit yourself only two stray pounds before you call a halt and you cancel all leaves of absence from your Tapered Eating. Two pounds are easily managed if you do something about them immediately. But if you let those two pounds hang around you for a while, they become a part of your figure. Then, as soon as your metabolism accommodates it, you will find two or three more pounds hanging on. Then once again you creep back to those old gymnastics of deception and guilt and the inevitable "depression eating," to make you feel better. Illogical logic!

Simply handle a quick two-pound weight gain as soon as it happens. Most normal-weight people contend with a few pounds time and again. Two pounds of prevention are worth buckets of cure. There also seems to be a close correlation between immediate remedy and frequency of recurrence. The problem disappears if it's deprived the strength of repetition.

Remember, your weight will change every day. Don't live on

the scale to control your behavior. The scale is not a home and your behavior is shaped by your purpose.

Your mind is the giant that directs your perception and your drive. Don't change your weight; change your mind, and your body will take shape.

With the Mannix Method, losing weight is only a by-product of gaining health. Obviously, when you regain lost weight, you have carelessly allowed your healthy, vital feeling of well-being to diminish. A Yo-Yo way of life is an unhealthy life-style. Build the foundation of your behavior with mature reason and a tornado won't affect you.

Your food choices have changed and your behavior has changed. You are trained, you are prepared, you are in control, you are responsible. Never forget the story of the superstar basketball player practicing easy sure shots hour after hour. Practice your basic skill, reinforce your attitude about food every time you see it. If you practice good behavior it becomes automatic. Life is too short and too exciting to be all wrapped up in fat. Enlarge your horizons. Focus your attention away from your mouth, become "other" directed, people oriented.

Complete this week. Use the Mannix Method as a reference book now that you have incorporated new behavior. Tapered Eating is your property as a basic eating procedure. Adjust the style to suit yourself, with your feelings and your scale to guide you. On your heavy days (no more than two pounds' worth) stick closely to Tapered Eating.

Whether you are eating Tapered style exactly or making amendments for special occasional occasions, eat nothing without thoughtfully considering the *procedure, implication,* and *consequences.* If you decide to eat something contrary to your training, be aware of it and enjoy it. Enjoy everything that you eat. Food and life are wonderful gifts.

51 HIGHLIGHTS

Fifty-one reminders follow. If you are one of those people who read the last part of a book first, and you have not lived the Mannix Method, please don't practice these techniques out of training

Commit yourself by signing the following contract.

Remember that this is a point of honor—a private obligation to yourself:

CONTRACT

With my initials below, I pledge my best effort in following each and every step in the Mannix Method described in Session _____12_____ for the next 7 days.

Initial: _____

Date: _____

context. Although they are precisely the methods used, the Mannix Method is a gradual *process training* that combines skill with time. There is nothing "instant," thoughtless, nor unnatural in this way of life.

1. **Tapered Eating.**

   Eat your largest meal at the start of the day. Eat your smallest meal at the end of the day.

2. **Take Thirty Minutes to Eat Every Meal** (never to be altered).

   Take small bites, replace the fork after every bite, sip water for interruption and pacing, chew slowly, and empty your mouth of each bite of food before taking the next.

3. **Take Two Intermissions.**

   Push yourself away from the table for one minute, twice. Take a deep breath each time to listen for your appestat.

4. **Eat Only At Designated Places.**

   Do not eat: standing, in the car, in bed, on the couch, or anyplace not designated for eating. Make this a hard-and-fast rule, never, never to be broken.

5. **Eat Only. Perform No Other Activity.**

   Do not watch television or talk on the telephone.
      (Reading is permitted, after the ninth week of training, but if you read and eat together, keep them separate.)

6. **Leave Two Bites.**

   Prepare too much if you must, and leave two bites on every plate. Do not run out of food.

7. **Make Unnecessary Food Inaccessible.**

   Store leftovers in opaque containers. Shelve snack foods like crackers or peanuts out of reach. Freeze as much extra food as you can. Buy only food that needs some preparation.

8. **Eat Deliberately. Make It Worth Your While.**

   Be aware of what you eat. Enjoy everything that you eat or don't eat it.

9. **Observe Good Table Manners.**

   Talk with your mouth empty and never with a fork in your hand. Talk some, eat some, but never at the same time. Good manners keep you thin, they are time-tested measures of control.

10. **Serve All Food From the Kitchen.**

    Keep serving platters off the table. Make it an effort to get more food.

11. **Make Eating Important.**

    Set attractive tables, prepare enticing plates. Ceremony makes eating more important. Ceremony provides for a less casual attitude.

12. **Never Skip Breakfast or Lunch.**

    These are absolutely necessary times to eat. Skip supper anytime you wish.

13. **Bank Calories.**

    Avoid it now to enjoy it later. Find taste-alikes. Eliminate unnecessary ingredients. Substitute when you can so you may enjoy those special foods later.

14. **Breathe to Eat.**

    Breathe deeply before meals; breathe deeply during meals at your intermissions, and breathe deeply after meals to relax your eating momentum. Breathe deeply whenever you want to alleviate tension. Breathe in, inflate your belly, hold for four seconds, then exhale for fifteen seconds.

15. **Don't Eat Anything for Thirty Minutes After a Meal.**
Give your appestat time to signal, then allow the motion of
eating to halt.

16. **Delay Starting Time.**
Delay starting to eat for one minute to allay any sense of time
emergency.

17. **Ten-Percent Maintenance Protects Your Investment.**
Five percent food management, five percent body management—two and a half hours a day.

18. **Twenty-One Days Builds a Habit.**
Twenty-one repetitions of an action develop a dependable
habit.

19. **Weigh Every Morning to Guide Eating.**
Get in shape, be in control, stray only two pounds. After you
have lost your extra weight, use the scale as a guide each
morning.

20. **Shop With a List, After Eating.**
Always market thirty minutes (at least) after eating. Delay
affects Why, What, and How much you buy.

21. **Intermittent Reinforcement Builds Strong Bad Habits.**
Do not occasionally reinforce old, out-of-control eating habits. You will build them into monsters.

22. **Get Out of Ruts. Change Rituals Often.**
Sameness begets boredom; boredom begets frustration; frustration begets distress; and distress requires coping. Shed ritual shelters—they aren't very protective.

23. **Look at Yourself Disrobed Daily in the Mirror.**
Twice is better, in the morning and again at night. Notice the
positive changes and recognize the negatives. Visualize the
real hidden you and tell yourself, aloud, that you like yourself.

24. **Plan Ahead.**
Don't invite surprise. Anticipate, plan, and implement.
Watch for situation recurrences.

25. **Eating Is the Problem, Not Food.**

26. **Relax.**
Practice relaxation techniques every day to make them effective.

27. **Keep Fluid Flowing.**
Don't force fluids, but know that your system needs a flow of liquids to stay healthy and to eliminate fat. No soft drinks, please.
28. **Restrict Caffeine.**
Caffeine is addictive, alters blood-sugar levels, causes depression, fatigue, and hunger.
29. **Alcohol Has Empty Calories.**
Alcohol is addictive and robs the body of valuable nutrients.
30. **Walk or Exercise One Hour Daily** (after completing training). Move to maintain life. Let exercise evolve from walking. Don't force it.
31. **Cheating Is a Childish Shelter.**
32. **There Are Four Inches From Chew to Swallow.**
Four inches of taste sensation, and you wear it.
33. **Don't Panic: Weight Fluctuates.**
Everyone's weight changes from day to day. Today's weight reflects three days of food intake and metabolic changes.
34. **Wait Thirty Minutes After Each Meal to Clean the Kitchen.**
Wind down to feel full to avoid nibbling.
35. **Forget Yourself.**
Don't think like a fat person. Revel in control and confidence instead.
36. **Take No Food for Four Hours Before Sleep.**
Food eaten less than four hours before sleep will become fat.
37. **Use Imaging to Snap Out of An Eating Trance.**
Involve your mind with more rewarding themes.
38. **Practice Flooding Before Eating Wrong Foods.**
Flood your thoughts with images that create unpleasant feelings. Repeat this when appropriate—it will soon be very effective.
39. **Life's Ups and Downs Won't End When You Are Thin.**
Know yourself. Establish realistic expectations. Life is always a series of problems that want solution.
40. **Before Snacking Try:**
Water, walking, relaxation, perfuming, bathing, brushing your teeth, writing a letter, etc., etc. Divert your attention, let the feeling pass.

41. **Understand "Food Days."**
    Unreasonable appetite is sometimes normal; "food days" are common experience. Eat more if you must, but only at meals.

42. **Learn to Read When You Eat Alone.**
    This advanced technique is a useful tool. Divide your time, eating and reading separately, together.

43. **Anticipate, Plan, Implement.**
    Review the procedure, the implications, and the consequences of every eating encounter.

44. **Food Management.**
    Intelligent food management must dictate the right time for the right food.

45. **Don't Fast to Lose Weight.**
    Fasting is a pleasant experience, with a doctor's permission. It is not a way to lose weight.

46. **Get Involved.**
    Stay busy and interested in the "other" guy and the world around you.

47. **Think Before You Act: That's Control.**

48. **Accept Yourself.**
    Perfection is not possible. Accept your imperfections.

49. **Change Is Part of Living.**

50. **Negative Thoughts Produce Negative Action.**

51. **Maturity Is the Ability to Give Up Some Things to Get Other Things.**

APPENDIX A

FOOD JOURNAL SAMPLE PAGE

Directions: Take this book to a photocopying machine and reproduce twenty (20) pages to be trimmed, stapled and used as a
booklet or inserted in a pocket checkbook cover.

DATE	START TIME	FOOD/AMOUNT	ATTITUDE	FINISH TIME	TOTAL EATING TIME

APPENDIX B

WEIGHT GRAPH

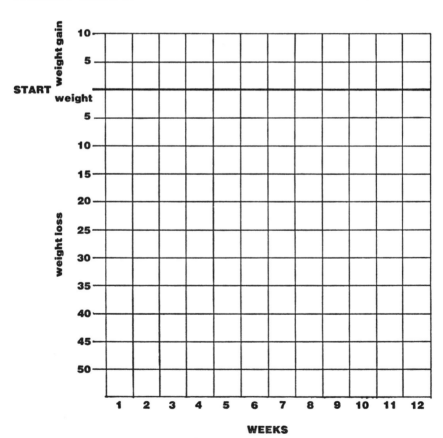

DIRECTIONS: Enter starting weight in blank space in left margin. *Weigh once a week only*. Record your weight with a dot above the week on training. Connect dots each week with a continuing unbroken line to indicate success of behavior change.